Wholly
Alive

You cannot help men permanently by doing for them what they could and should do for themselves.
　　　　　　　—Abraham Lincoln

Treat people as if they were what they ought to be and you help them become what they are capable of being.
　　　　　　　—Johann W. von Goethe

Wholly Alive

Richard Kaplan, D.O.
Barry Saltzman, D.O.
Laurence Ecker, D.O.
with
Patrick Wilkins

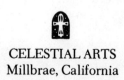

CELESTIAL ARTS
Millbrae, California

Celestial Arts
231 Adrian Road
Millbrae, California 94030

Cover design by Abigail Johnston
Cover photograph by Lance Cepuder

First Printing March 1979

Made in the United States of America

Library of Congress Cataloging in Publication Data

Saltzman, Barry, 1944–
    Wholly alive.

        Bibliography: p.
        1. Health.   2. Mind and body.   I. Kaplan,
Richard, 1945–   joint author.   II. Ecker,
Laurence, 1949–   joint author.   III. Title.
RA776.5.S24   613   78-67852
ISBN 0-89087-237-6

1 2 3 4 5 6 7 — 85 84 83 82 81 80 79

Contents

Dedication

To our patients,
past, present and future.
whose needs we strive to serve.

Acknowledgments

We sincerely express our thanks and appreciation to Janice Gregory for her unstinting efforts in the transcription of tapes and the typing and retyping of manuscript pages in the preparation of this book.

Our gratitude also goes out to the staff at all the Holistic Medical Group clinics for their valuable practical contributions.

Introduction

It is now well recognized that the major determinants of health are nutrition, physical exercise and mental attitude; the latter is perhaps the most important, for it contributes to use of nutrition and physical exercise! If each individual would only follow the simple, basic instructions for good health as outlined in *Wholly Alive*, practicing basically good nutrition, exercising regularly and using a positive attitude in creating a positive lifestyle, it would do more good for the health of people in this country than all the physicians, drugs, hospitals and surgery in the history of the world. The next step really is up to *you!* Books such as *Wholly Alive* can help you know which way to turn to help create your own health. I would emphasize, however, that reading is of no value if you don't practice it!

Best wishes in creating your own health.

C. Norman Shealy, M.D., Ph.D.
Founder and Senior Dolorologist, Pain and Health Rehabilitation Center;
Author of *90 Days to Self-Health*, *The Pain Game*, and *Occult Medicine Can Save Your Life*;
President of the American Holistic Medical Association

Foreword

How do you view medicine today? Probably the first thought that springs to mind is sickness. Developing that a little, you would no doubt move on to doctors, prescriptions, pills, hospitals and clinics, until you had built up a picture of health care as it exists in the second half of this century.

There is, however, evidence now emerging that our basic ideas and beliefs are changing. A health care revolution is taking place which concerns you and everyone around you. As doctors, we believe it will have such a profound effect that it will change completely your concept of medical treatment. If you are asked that same question—How do you view medicine?—ten years from now, you will probably think not of sickness, doctors, hospitals and pills, but of *me, my body, my mind, my state of well-being.* The medicine of the very near future is going to emphasize *prevention* of illness rather than treatment.

This is the only commonsense long-term solution to a present-day medical system that both inadequately serves the people and threatens them with a tide of ever-rising costs. It

1

already sets the country back a million dollars an *hour* just to keep the service going; and government economists have calculated that annual health care costs in the United States could soar above the $200 billion mark annually before this decade is out. What's more, these costs are going up more than two and one-half times faster than anything else in the economy, and at that rate, the figure of $200 billion could double within five years. By the year 2000, estimates the National Institute of Health, total costs will be $1 *trillion*.

What does that mean to you? It means higher taxes and insurance premiums. But more important, it means you may soon have to start making choices about health care over the other necessities and pleasures of life. *It could soon get too expensive to be ill.*

What is at fault is the approach to health. Doctors will do their utmost to find cures for ills like cancer, heart disease and every illness known. No matter how rare the disease, there is always some physician somewhere, ready to meet the challenge. People will always talk about the "miracles" our hospitals achieve and we never stop hearing about heart transplants and other spectacular milestones of medical "progress." But these technological feats are not really moving us forward in our goal of good health. They are simply combatting the effects of bad health.

This type of health care is known within medical circles as "after-the-fact" medicine; that is, it functions when there has been a crisis. You become ill first and then the doctor steps in.

But, as we know, this system is expensive. It is not conducive to long life either. The average age at which American men and women die has hardly changed in more than half a century. Life expectancy for people who reach the age of fifty-five has increased only two years since 1900. That is rather sad when doctors, patients, politicians and administrators alike boast that this country has the best health care in the world.

Clearly the door is open for change, just as the noted French physician Descartes saw room for improvement when he revolutionized medical care in the seventeenth century, dividing the person into mind and body, laying the groundwork for specialization. In time, plagues, typhoid, diphtheria and other now virtually forgotten diseases were no longer mysteries as physicians everywhere championed a glorious age of discovery. They all went forward until today's serious illnesses, already mentioned, presented their respective challenges.

In the meantime however, differences in the way the American people live their lives have occurred. Everyone has a car, a comfortable, centrally heated home, convenience and junk food, chemically treated tap water; the lifestyle of the tough and hardy American pioneers has changed to modern comfort and ease, a crucial transition.

We have been making ourselves sicker and sicker. So much so, that apart from the serious diseases we now have to cope with, we have also created a society of *moderately* ill people . . . not in enough trouble to go to hospital, but still sick enough to need regular visits to the doctor and a host of home remedies and prescription medicines.

These are people with chronic illnesses, and most chronic illnesses are preventable. In fact, three out of every four "sick" people have chronic diseases that could be prevented.

Holistic doctors base their philosophy on that one word—*prevention*. They focus on health, which is really the goal of all doctors, rather than on disease. But what is new is the way holistic doctors achieve that objective, by taking the emphasis for fighting illness away from drugs, surgery and hospitals, and putting it on the individual patient's ability to keep himself healthy. Holistic doctors acknowledge all the forms of medical treatment available today, but they prefer more natural therapies which correct the body's chemistry and stimulate its own defenses against illness. They are very much aware of them all.

This book describes this system of natural therapies. But like any system, it is only as good as the people who follow it. Above all, the desire to be as free from illness as possible must lie in the patient. All people, providing they are prepared to change their lifestyles to be more compatible with the demands of their bodies and minds, will benefit.

We all live in an environment of negative input, much of which is hard to avoid. Air pollution, sedentary lives because of the authomobile, high levels of stress in day-to-day activity, are integral parts of the business of living. The practice of holistic health helps people deal with these unhealthy factors and attempts to stimulate the body's own healing powers. The patient is seen as a whole person, ideally as one in balance with his environment and social circumstances. Using the holistic system, thousands of people who have been through our clinics have gotten their chronic illnesses under control.

Basically, good nutrition, exercise and stress management are the vehicles to good health. If you are prepared to change your life to include these, then the results are there for the taking. Obviously, if you want to smoke, eat junk food, or sit in front of the tube with your TV dinner night after night, then the system is not for you. But if you have the courage to take responsibility and demand something different, to demand good health and wellbeing,   then you can join the people who have already changed their lives and discovered a better way.

Life's Hangover

It's an ungodly hour in the morning. The alarm clock rings. You peer through the half-darkness of the bedroom, but your eyelids will hardly open to focus on the numbers. Through the mistiness you see the clock really is telling the truth—it's time to get up. But you don't want to. You could quit your job, anything to stay there a little longer, still numbed by sleep.

Slowly you force your body to move, push back the covers and ease yourself free. Your bedmate slumbers on. You don't whisper sweetly, "Wake up, darling," you grunt or shake a shoulder, mumbling something about the time. The thought of another day really hurts. The sourness in your stomach hits you. The fusty taste on your tongue makes you aware that you're breathing and uttering through a mouth contaminated by too much drink or smoke or food the night before.

You creak to your feet. Your back aches. Your legs are stiff. You straighten your shoulders, stretching dry fingers over your hipbones. Your joints appreciate the movements as they click into place and you reach for the bathrobe behind the door. Fumbling, you find the light switch; the 60-watt bulb seems like a spotlight as it blinds your eyes. You cover them momentarily and mutter, feeling your aches and pains again. They are your companions to the kitchen as you tell yourself reassuringly that you'll be okay when you've had your first cup of coffee.

But first you must clean your teeth to get rid of the taste in your mouth, right? You turn back from the kitchen and grope for the light in the bathroom. The daily routine starts. Toothbrush . . . toothpaste . . . squeeze . . . cold minty feeling . . . brush . . . arm almost dead with the motion . . . mouthful of water . . . squirt into the basin . . . dry with the towel. That's a little better, you think, but the coffee will do the trick. Good strong coffee. Though sometimes you have tea. Good strong tea. "Strong? Why do I always have it strong?" you ask yourself. Yes, that's right, it's the caffeine these doctors talk about. You know vaguely about that. But still, you like it. It doesn't do any harm and it does wake you up. It's life-giving liquid. It gets rid of that awful taste. It fills your body with energy. And you should know. After all, you've been doing it for years.

It's five minutes since you got out of bed . . . you return to the kitchen. The kettle has water in it from yesterday, so you fill it up from the tap. You put it on the stove and soon that cheerful steam is tumbling from the spout. The water gurgles as you pour it into the cup; the coffee swirls to white as you add the milk. You take a sip. Mmm, tastes good. The uplifting effect is almost immediate. A lump more sugar makes it even better. Cigarettes?—They're on the table. Of course, you always have a pack and matches on the table. It saves hunting through clothes you had on the day before. You pull one from the pack, light it and draw the smoke down deep into your lungs. At last your body is coming to life. Great, isn't it? That first cigarette of the morning. What a pleasure. Draw in more smoke . . . right down inside, then back up again, half through the nose, half through the mouth. The aches and pains are easing. . .

You finish the cigarette, shower, dress and it's half an hour since that rude alarm rang. Now the stiffness in your body has gone. You're ready for the day. . . . But you must remember to see the doctor sometime about that nagging little stomachache you always get at this time. Or perhaps it is a tight chest that the cough from your cigarette smoking clears. It might even be your asthma, your migraine or your constipation. You might have a sneaking suspicion of ulcers, or a weak heart that makes you breathless easily. It may even be your arthritis that seems to stay with you all day, all week or all month . . . continually, whether you're at work or relaxing.

Funny—have you noticed how you always say it's *yours* when you talk about illness? It's *"my* this, *my* that, *my* the other," whenever you mention it or think about it. It belongs to you. You live with it. You always have it.

It is called a "chronic" illness and it is what this book is all about. It is chronic because it keeps occurring, over and over again. It is not a crisis illness such as a broken bone, a stroke, a heart attack, an auto accident, a cancer discovered or a sudden disease that happens then heals. Chronic illnesses are clawing, nagging illnesses—nondescript at times, more specific at others—but always there.

You probably wonder why you get them and likely as not put it down to "getting on in years." You do? Well, there is no mystery about it, and if you have chronic illnesses, there's no reason why you must go on living with them. You do not have to wake up each morning with that bad taste in your mouth. You do not have to need coffee, cigarettes or a drink to feel active and alive. You do not have to take another lump of sugar to get some energy, or a hot shower to ease your aching joints.

It does not matter whether you are thirty, forty, fifty, sixty, seventy, or older. There is a way that you can get relief from chronic illnesses and aches and pains forever. It is called *holistic medicine* and it is not so much a treatment as a new way of life, because it uses *you* to fight the illness, rather than the vast arsenal of drugs and medications that most doc-

tors now dispense to do the same thing. These drugs and medications only mask the symptoms of illnesses temporarily.
They do not get to the root of your problems. With holistic
medicine, the whole of you is looked at in treating illnesses;
not just your aching arm or leg, but your entire person—
body, mind, environment and way of living—in order to
make you as free from sickness as possible.

The word *holistic* is derived from *holos* which translates
from the Greek as "whole"—all of you, body and mind.
Years ago, before the modernization of medicine, doctors
looked at people as a whole. There were few who specialized
as doctors do now, treating separately different parts of the
body. What specialization has achieved is admirable, but the
great majority of us never get to the stage where we need that
sort of specialization. Most of us get not severe, but chronic
illnesses. Yet the vast resources of money in our country's
health services are being plowed into crisis illnesses and spe-
cializations. Something is clearly wrong. Why not place the
emphasis on *preventing* illness instead?

The Holistic Doctor

You are probably wondering by now just how did traditional doctors such as ourselves, trained at medical schools, actually make the transition from the present health care system to holistic medicine?

It goes back to our starting medical school. Like all would-be doctors, we had made a decision to devote our lives to caring for people. We realized that by learning from a vast field of knowledge going back centuries we would be performing a public service.

Looking back, it would appear that we must have been something approaching renegades, although we didn't think so at the time. We were just as dedicated to our cause as the others, but something kindled an interest in alternative therapies . . . therapies like nutrition and stress management that were outside the spectrum of medical school training. Gradually, we began to feel that the medicine we were being taught did not have all the answers, and we had to search for different ways to fill the gaps in our knowledge. We worked and qualified within the medical establishment, but we never forgot the doctors who influenced us most in those early years. It was they who, with their courage to seek out nontoxic treatments (many of which we now use in our clinics), sowed the seeds.

Gradually, those newer treatments mingled with our traditional knowledge. It was an accumulative process, for you cannot learn two or three alternative methods then rush out and practice them. It has to be much fuller, with substantial amounts from both sides of the medical "tree." We are trying to incorporate what we think are the most worthwhile and strongest points of traditional medicine with the new approaches we have studied and believe to be important. It is the cream of the old with the cream of the new.

Above all, we are striving to prevent illness; to preserve and maintain the quality of life that we think everyone should be experiencing.

AN OUNCE OF PREVENTION IS WORTH A POUND OF CURE

Ask yourself: When was the last time you were a patient in a hospital? Probably never, maybe once or twice. You would be in an even smaller minority if the technical and sophisticated resources of modern medical care had ever saved your life.

This is a fact: Even if you don't need the facilities, you work several weeks of every year just to make your contribution to the nation's health bill through taxes and insurance premiums. It is getting worse by the day, with costs rising at about twice the rate of inflation. Skyrocketing prices in the "getting well" business could rise to $1 trillion dollars by the year 2000. Much of the present $180 billion annually is going to pay the medical staff of the system. There are some 400,000 doctors in 7000 hospitals and clinics. They have one million nurses and more than two million health workers to help them. There are 125 medical schools to be supported, some of them through the drug companies which are themselves a billion-dollar-a-year industry. All these are growing rapidly, along with their payrolls. And then there's the hardware. But to what end?

Any sensible American, if he works it out for himself, will see that the Department of Health, Education and Welfare, which publicly gasps over the figures, is not just toying with rapidly multiplying numbers. The problem is real and of monstrous proportions, and those in medical and health administrative circles keep saying they are concerned at the sharply upward trend of costs, yet few brakes are applied and the spending goes on. In hospitals, federal economists report, there is a "keeping up with the Joneses" attitude every time a new piece of medical equipment comes on the market. One example of the very latest is the Computerized Axial Tomograph, or CAT scanner (an ultra-sophisticated form of X-ray equipment) for which a hospital is paid extra money, by an insurance company, every time it is used. Many hospitals have them installed at a cost of half a million dollars each. If every general hospital in the country gets one, three billion dollars will have been spent.

If you go to the hospital with a headache you could be given the benefit of a "CAT scan." Yet, in most cases, a headache has a simple cause. The CAT scanner is a great piece of equipment, but not necessary in every hospital, and technological advancement is likely to make it obsolete within a short period of time.

Now this, you may say, is none of your concern because the insurance company, or Medicare/Medicaid, pays. That attitude, unfortunately, has led us to believe that getting health care in the United States is like drawing water from a tap; so much so that you do not hope, but *expect* a cure if you get ill. You have been conditioned to believe that health care is there at your disposal. It is this "grab and take" free-for-all that places the enormous demands on the system. One eminent and concerned physician said it this way: "If we sold cars the way we sell health in the United States, everyone would have a Rolls Royce." A nice thought, but economic madness!

Common sense tells us that preventing illness is a far better long-term solution to today's situation. In the fields of heart disease and cancer, this is already being done, but in comparison to traditional "defensive" medicine the amount of money being spent on across-the-board prevention is minimal—only 1 percent of health care dollars.

Little or nothing outside the work of holistic health is being done about the remaining chronic illnesses. Somehow, the adage "an ounce of prevention is worth a pound of cure" has gotten lost in the life, death and dollars equation that is now American health care.

A BETTER WAY

Holistic doctors took a new look at this problem and saw that if illness is to be permanently prevented the patient must accept some responsibility for his own health. To put that simply: you must become the doctor and we, the doctors, must become the teachers. Education is the key word. You must learn and, perhaps for the first time in your life, be aware of what your body needs and doesn't need to survive in this world.

There is no magic in medicine and there is no mystery about being well or getting on the road to good health. To do it you need only understand the aims, objectives and thinking behind holistic health and put the lessons into practice on yourself.

Although holistic medicine is emerging now, it is not new. Indeed, it is the type of medicine that has its roots in many cultures throughout the world, past and present. It is only in the last few hundred years that medicine has become fragmented into specialties, and then only in what we know as the Western World of North America and Europe.

When physicians had fewer tools at their disposal, all diagnosis was done by direct observation. It was seen instantly that there were connections between the patient's physical, psychological and environmental circumstances, and that all of them may have been influencing the illness. Yet it is impossible under today's medical care system to get complete attention to your problems without consulting a psychiatrist, a public health expert, a general practitioner, an internist, a nutritionist and a host of other specialists.

Holistic medicine simplifies all that. Holistic doctors set out specifically to deal in all those areas at once. This is not just another specialization, but a realization that it is the only commonsense way of dealing with chronic illness.

Good health is the state in which the body functions at its best. A fully functional person therefore has no symptoms such as headaches, colds, or constipation, and can live free of the remedies constantly being thrust upon us by radio, television and newspaper advertising. Such a person has all the energy necessary to fulfill normal activities during the course of a day. We all know such people and enviously notice that they rarely get depressed or anxious and always have a sense of well-being and relaxation. This is because their body chemistry functions correctly. The rest of us must contend with these basic enemies:

- **Genetic vulnerability.** Many of us have inborn deficiencies which expose us to chronic illness from the start.
- **Environmental insults.** Pollution, lack of sunshine, tap water with chemical additives, poor living conditions all weaken our natural defenses, both physical and psychological.
- **Lowered resistance.** A result of poor nutrition, lack of exercise, and inability to deal with environmental insults.

Modern medical care offers only drugs and surgery to correct imbalances within the body. Holistic doctors recommend natural methods, employing drugs and surgery only as last resorts. From HMG (Holistic Medical Group) clinics alone, thousands of people ill with chronic diseases have been made better when all other forms of traditional therapy have failed. You simply have to be prepared to abandon lifelong, deeply ingrained habits which may be making you ill.

A big part of the holistic treatment is to educate you, the patient, in wise food choice to enable intake of only those foods good for your body. In this country, before the days of frozen and processed food, little was done to make food look or taste better than it actually was. Mom spent her days in the kitchen, baking and cooking, using virtually all fresh foods. Vegetables were grown in the backyard and Dad picked them on the day they were to be eaten. Though he probably didn't know it, the fresh vegetables he picked contained all the food fiber and vitamins his family needed. Yet today, the majority of people in this country eat few fresh vegetables; they are mostly canned or frozen, both of which processes seriously deplete their nutritional value.

These types of vegetables are preferred because they are quicker and more convenient to prepare. But as a general guideline, anything, not only vegetables, that has to be prepared for you in a package or a can may be bad for the body. Processed food, even if it has few chemical additives, is of less nutritional value than fresh food and its long-term use may be a significant contributory factor to chronic illness. It is because of this that holistic patients are gradually weaned away from processed foods to a more natural diet.

Relief from illness cannot happen overnight. It is necessary to see the bad habits that contribute to chronic illness— not only poor nutrition, but lack of exercise, excessive stress and exposure to pollution—and decide to adopt a whole new lifestyle. If you can do that, then you can work towards avoiding the illness crisis. Most illness is a sign of previous neglect or abuse of your body. If this can be corrected naturally, rather than by symptom-relieving drugs, genuine prevention can take place. But the solution lies with you, and you alone, because you have to learn how and why your body works the way it does so that natural, inner healing can take place. It's a big responsibility to take your health into your own hands, but it can and will bring results, if you really want it to. Think of it in terms of this old adage: "You can give a hungry man a fish and he'll be satisfied, But teach that same man to fish for himself and he'll never be hungry again."

That is holistic health in a nutshell. More and more, traditional doctors, tired of dispensing the same prescription time and again to the same patients, are changing to the holistic way to prevent future illness. Modern medical care, it cannot be denied, has been excellent in treating acute clinical cases like broken limbs, fractures and wounds, but has failed in dealing with chronic illness.

Holistic doctors on many occasions refrain from administering painkillers and anti-inflammatory medications, using natural methods of treatment instead. Nervous people and insomniacs who had been treated with traditional pills have been encouraged to adopt a holistic lifestyle and have enjoyed good health without all the side effects of drugs. They are able to throw out their Valium, Dalmane and phenobarbital.

Thomas Edison seemed to understand the concept of holistic health perfectly when he forecast years ago: "The doctor of the future will prescribe no drugs, but will interest his patient in the care and nutrition of the human frame and in the cause and prevention of disease."

COMPLETING THE HANGOVER CYCLE

Before we proceed further toward achieving a holistic lifestyle, think back for a moment to our character of the first few pages who had difficulty getting up in the morning. The scenario was set up to illustrate the way chronic disease becomes a part of living—as a permanent hangover—and it's worth developing just a little.

We left him dressed, ready for work and about to go to his car. He could certainly have walked a mile to catch a bus to his office, and if he were really aware of the value of exercise he most certainly would have. For he, like the majority of Americans, is up to 30 percent above his ideal weight. Needless to say, he does not walk. It's so much easier by car, as you might know, even though it's always a hassle to park. It's the same every morning, with a buildup of frustration and stress as colleagues arriving earlier take the best spots in the lot.

But he makes it just in time. "Good morning," sound the cheery voices around him. He doesn't reply. All he can think about is that he needs food to stop the acid feeling in his stomach.

"A bacon and egg sandwich, please, Miss Smith," goes the coffee break order. Coffee break? He's only just arrived. Of course, he needs coffee to keep him going.

"Those reports still need doing," our character sighs to himself. The tension is mounting again. Hands are sweating. Blood pressure is rising. The telephone rings. He'll call back . . . headache . . . aspirin . . . the reports . . . gulp . . . sandwich . . . another coffee . . . cigarette . . . noon . . . need a drink . . . the reports. . . .

Wait! Everybody has to take a lunch break, he reasons. It's the only sane part of the day, the time to unwind the tension, the time to get into the bar across the street. It's all the boys together and costs a lot of money. Still, two or three strong bourbons and a deli sandwich with a beer to wash it down are welcome, and it's good for planning and strategy to talk in the bar over lunch.

Two hours later he takes the elevator up three floors to start the afternoon. He could walk up the stairs—it's only three flights. But the breathlessness, remember. It's the same with interoffice visits—always either the elevator or the intercom system. It's easier and quicker; he's a busy man and *time is money.*

There's no end to the tension. This time it's the traffic at the end of the working day. The rush hour. The freeway is murderous. Our tensed-up character is easily annoyed and becomes frustrated when the traffic slows to a crawl.

Finally he gets home. Relief shows in his face as he puts his car in the garage for the night. The thought of that steak and french fries waiting for him makes him feel good. The warmth of the house pleasantly engulfs him as he opens the door.

Then, that routine again . . . the armchair . . . the TV news . . . the steak, thick and juicy . . . the after-dinner cigarette (the best of the day) . . . the coziness of the living room . . . the eight o'clock movie . . . the cool beer. All thoughts of tomorrow's stress are gone, buried in the late-night talk show. His lot is sweet oblivion after a salami sandwich, as our fat, balding, red-faced friend slips into the slumber that will leave him just as miserable tomorrow.

Now you may think he is an extreme example of someone who suffers from chronic diseases. He is not. In fact, he is a perfect model of the find of person the past twenty-five years of fast living, convenience foods, automobiles and affluence have brought about. He is very much Mr. Average and he is slowly killing himself by his own hand. A thorough doctor's examination would no doubt find that his symptoms are related to his faulty lifestyle.

GETTING BETTER

The first question you must ask yourself in getting better is: "How good—or bad—do I feel now?" It is probably difficult for you to answer, because most people take chronic illness and their way of life for granted. Often they spare little thought to what they are doing, why they do it, or the consequences of an ache here and a pain there.

To help you carry out what is probably the first honest health evaluation of yourself, the HMG devised the following *Feeling Good Scale*—a lifestyle quality indicator—so that you can see where you stand on the health ladder.

THE FEELING GOOD SCALE

100% OPTIMAL HEALTH. People born with good constitutions. Can fight many diseases. Lots of energy. Relaxed, free from symptoms. Need neither alcohol nor drugs to make them feel good. Follow good diet and exercise regularly.

90% GOOD HEALTH. Rarely depressed or anxious. No personality problems, though looking to improve themselves through regular exercise, good diet, yoga, etc. Have occasional headaches or "off" day.

80% People free of illness who generally find life rewarding. Occasional alcohol or drugs give mild temporary kick but are of no significance. Rare visits to the doctor. Occasional cold, headaches, bout of the blues or personal problem. Takes occasional exercise, follows fairly good diet.

70% MEDIUM HEALTH. Has poor diet, doesn't exercise. Has acne, excessively dry/oily hair or skin, dandruff. Prone to colds. Has cravings for chocolate, sweets, cookies, cakes, coffee, tea, cigarettes, or snacks of favorite food. Overweight. High blood pressure. Frequent anxiety, stress. Lacks energy. Depressed often. Has in excess of three glasses of beer, wine or soft drinks every day. Regular use of home remedies advertised on TV. Plagued by allergies, nervousness, flu, insomnia, obesity, tension headaches, poor memory, infections, irritability, migraine, palpitations, ulcers, asthma, arthritis, heart disease, constant aches and pains. Eats processed and convenience foods (frozen or canned). High meat and carbohydrate consumption. Needs salt. Uses sweeteners to enhance food tastes.

30% POOR HEALTH. Takes pills and medications every day. Cardiovascular, gastrointestinal, psychiatric illnesses. Heavy alcohol drinkers.

20% CLINICALLY ILL. These people have lost the ability to help themselves, Need surgery, medical or psychiatric supervision.

10% CRITICALLY ILL.

0% DEAD.

Having studied the scale, you will now be aware of the pitfalls of some of today's lifestyles. Use it only as a general guide to the level at which you function. It will help you if it simply points out a few bad habits that make you less healthy than you could be. But don't let that be yet another burden to bear. Just the opposite. Look upon it as an awareness that something is wrong. If you can do that, you have already taken the first step toward a new life.

If you are like the majority of chronically ill individuals, you will have placed yourself on the scale somewhere between the 40 and 70 percent marks. You are in medium health and there are millions like you, with general aches and pains kept in control by home remedies and prescription drugs. Adopt the new lifestyle of all holistic patients, however, and you could spring right up into the good health category. Often it is difficult to get people up to 100 percent optimal health because of inborn factors partially controlling illness. But by following the rules, you could rise in dramatic fashion. How long it takes depends largely on how long you have had your problem or problems and how severe they are. It may take only three months to see an improvement; then again, it could take a year. The time limit, though, is not important because permanent changes are going to be instituted. You cannot rush the course of holistic medicine.

Deeply entrenched bad habits from a whole lifetime cannot be changed overnight. Much of it is relearning how to live and, as with any learning process, you must take it step by step, in order that it be retained.

THE HOLISTIC VIEW OF CHRONIC ILLNESS

Holistic doctors believe that knowledge of the chronic diseases is not widespread among ordinary people because many physicians will not discuss with the patient the causes of their ills. This occurs, partly, because medicine is a highly complicated subject; answering your questions simply takes more time than most traditional doctors have. As the holistic doctor is more of a teacher, he believes it is his duty to pass on the knowledge that his profession has given him. For that reason, this chapter is devoted to describing the causes and symptoms of some of the most common chronic illnesses. These descriptions will prepare you to start the fight against illness.

Cardiovascular Disorders

The heart is the body's engine, a pump constantly pushing blood through the arteries and veins; hence, chronic disorders of the heart are termed "cardiovascular" (*cardio*, heart, and *vascular*, blood vessels). It's like the engine and transmission of an automobile, absolutely vital to the efficient running of the car. But just like the engine of a car, the heart needs to be kept in good condition if it is to remain useful; and unfortunately, just like most engines, it frequently is not. In fact, most people remain totally unaware of its "servicing" needs. Like cars running on the wrong type of gasoline, owners give it the wrong types of fuel. While the heart really appreciates a balanced, nutritious diet, most people feed on fatty foods that serve only to clog the blood vessels with a substance called *cholesterol*. Second, like a car kept in the garage unused, they keep the body inactive. The heart doesn't like that any more than the car engine, because exercise is vital to its continued running. Third, an automobile performs far better when it is driven gently without quick stops and starts which cause strain to the engine. In other words, like the human heart, too much stress doesn't do it much good.

So there are three ways in which the average heart is misused. Little wonder that cardiovascular disorders account for more than 50 percent of deaths in the United States. It almost seems as though, like most automobiles, scrapping after a certain number of years is perfectly acceptable. But is it? Holistic doctors suspect many people simply do not look upon heart death as being preventable, but accept that certain types of people die of heart attacks. It is acknowledged that there are many different ways that heart attacks can occur apart from wrong diet, too little exercise and stress. But these are the main causes and they *can* be prevented.

That is why cardiovascular disorders are a major concern of holistic health care. In fact, holistic doctors believe that just about everybody in the United States has incipient heart disease. The question is, to what degree?

The heart diseases most prevalent in the American people are *atherosclerosis* (buildups of cholesterol inside the arteries, constricting the flow of blood) and *arteriosclerosis* (a thickening or hardening of the arteries), which affect the heart's good functioning. They can exist for years unnoticed, but eventually the body gives out warning signs such as pains in the chest, left arm or leg, and these should be heeded, for the consequences of inattention can be fatal. These pains could come after an exertion of, say, running for a bus. They're most likely to happen if you're over thirty-five years old, thirty pounds or so above your normal weight, smoke and get little exercise. Even if you recognize only a couple of the traits in yourself, you could still come into the risk category, so do not be complacent. Also do not get into the chronic illness pattern of living with chest pains, putting

them off as insignificant. They are warning signals, which if
acted upon early enough could prevent your untimely death.

Finally, for all doubters: Just remember when you stand
back in admiration of the wonderful rescue work now being
achieved by this nation's cardiologists in emergency wards
from New York to Los Angeles . . . about two-thirds of all
heart attack victims are *dead before* they reach the hospital.

Hypertension or High Blood Pressure

Connected with cardiac disease, the link is that everybody
who has it will eventually have signs of heart disease; but not
everyone with heart disease, of course, has hypertension. You
might be surprised to know high blood pressure is at epidemic proportions in this country. Some 20,000,000 people have
it, although it's estimated that only 50 percent of them actually know it. It's a condition that is treated by the present
medical care system with anti-hypertensive drugs and low-
salt diets, which are helpful in many cases.

Holistic doctors, however, look at other factors and contributing causes like overweight, stress, heavy coffee drinking
and even air pollution in an attempt to reduce the need for
medication. In fact, according to a study carried out by doctors at the Western Infirmary in Glasgow, Scotland, successful weight loss has a "significant" correlation with decreased
blood pressure.

How can you tell if you are one of those people who have
high blood pressure and don't know it? A good way is to
check your blood pressure at any of the public machines you
find in shopping malls, clinics, etc. For a few cents, you at-
tach the test cuff to your arm and get a reading within
minutes. A normal reading should be around 120 over 80,
indicating the pressure when the heart is beating (120) and
when it is relaxed (80). If it is over those figures, then it is
time to take preventive measures before symptoms like headaches, dizziness and blurred vision become apparent.

Rheumatoid Arthritis

Despite its familiarity to most people, arthritis is still something of a mystery to medical researchers because what causes it is not fully understood. It is what is known as a *systemic* (that is, of the body's whole system, rather than a localized disorder) disease which, as you've probably seen by the incidence among friends and relatives, affects more women than men. In fact, the figure is three times more female than male sufferers, and they're usually over 25. It's painful, too. Most sufferers have no doubt that they've got it. For those who may be unknowingly experiencing the early stages of arthritis, it's time to start checking when even slight pains occur in the joints (particularly hands or feet) accompanied by tiredness and possibly early morning stiffness or discomfort. Another early sign is a once smooth-fitting ring that now seems difficult to slide off the finger; it's those middle finger joints where arthritis sufferers can also be affected by swelling. Aspirin is used to some effect, as well as steroids which may help to reduce the inflammation. Holistic doctors, however, prefer to treat it differently initially, using improved nutrition, exercise, checking for food allergies and hormone imbalances before using other therapies, such as chelation or medication.

Carbohydrate Intolerance

This is the name given to adult-onset diabetes and hypoglycemia, although most doctors would describe the latter as a symptom rather than a disease. Diabetes, however, is very much an illness and it affects in varying degrees some 10,000,000 Americans of all ages and both sexes.

It is referred to as a carbohydrate intolerance because that is what happens when the body cannot utilize carbohydrate foods in the normal way. When a nondiabetic eats foods like bread, rice, potatoes, sugar and candy, a hormone called insulin is produced by the pancreas to allow the sugar, into which all carbohydrate is converted, to be utilized by the body. Diabetics, however, either cannot produce the necessary amount of insulin or it cannot be utilized. Until they get on a course of treatment, diabetics find they must consume more and more food to satisfy excessive hunger and thirst, which results in excessive urination as the unfortunate sufferer gets caught up in a vicious circle.

The most obvious way to control the symptoms is to introduce insulin artificially into the body, and this many diabetics do through self-injections with a hypodermic syringe. Coupled with that, a diabetic must follow a special diet restricting refined carbohydrate and fat.

Doctors agree that there is a hereditary predisposition to the disease; holistic doctors *emphasize* that if a person begins as early as possible a diet low in refined carbohydrates and fats he is less likely to develop the symptoms of adult onset diabetes.

It is here that the diagnosis of hypoglycemia becomes significant, because most sufferers from hypoglycemia are likely to become diabetic if they continue with a similar diet of excessive sugar and carbohydrates. Holistic doctors believe hypoglycemia to be so widespread that 50 percent of the people in this country have it, although of course, in the vast majority it remains undiagnosed. (On more than one occasion, holistic doctors have found these patients inappropriately treated with tranquilizers or referred to psychiatrists.) Hypoglycemia occurs as a result of excess sugar consumption, and it puts a constant strain on the adrenal glands and the pancreas. This can produce symptoms such as loss of memory, confusion, hallucinations, fatigue, headaches, sweating, low blood pressure and even coma.

Often a person with hypoglycemia will feel tired a couple of hours after eating a meal. This is because eating has increased the blood sugar; the pancreas, which has produced the insulin, has been overstimulated; the insulin then lowers the blood sugar and the body becomes fatigued. So the next time you settle down with that after-meal sleepiness, think what it may mean. You could be consuming too much sugar and be hypoglycemic.

The average American is eating around 120 pounds of sugar every year, while 100 years ago Americans ate practically none. Why sugar consumption has risen so much is hard to say. It is probably a combination of advertising by the food industry and the fact that sugar is cheap and appeals to many people's tastes. It is also due to cultural encouragement. Since infancy, sugar, in the form of candy or chocolate, has meant a reward; all forms of thanks have assumed a sugary disposition.

Clearly, we all need to reduce our intake of sugar; it doesn't do us *any* good at all. The best way to stop using it is to take it off your table; then start looking at the processed foods and drinks containing sugar you may not have even been aware of before, such as all beer, spirits, sodas, cakes, cereals, breads, jams and sauces.

From the holistic casebook:

Oliver is a 30-year-old real estate salesman who sought help in a last ditch attempt to save his job. He had progressively been having extreme fatigue with episodes of disorientation and poor memory, and had been threatened by his employers with being fired. Furthermore, his wife had been unsympathetic towards his continual complaining and poor physical status and was on the brink of ending the marriage. A thorough examination was performed which included elaborate blood testing and a glucose tolerance test. The patient presented a normal glucose curve for the first three hours of the test, after which his glucose plummeted. This caused an exacerbation of his complaints. Upon questioning it was found that these symptoms did, in fact, arise after he was forced to go more than two hours without eating, and in fact, his diet had consisted predominantly of refined carbohydrates, candy bars and alcohol. This poor food intake had caused a hills-and-valleys effect in his blood sugar levels, the poor memory and disorientation being linked to the "valleys" and a euphoric, hyperactive state to the "hills." A diagnosis of reactive hypoglycemia was established. He was then placed on a diet consisting of protein, unprocessed vegetables and some fruits. He was instructed to carry a readily accessible natural food, such as nuts, to prevent those plummeting episodes of his blood sugar levels. These were to be consumed at intervals no greater than two hours. Oliver was also instructed to eat light amounts of food at each sitting so as not to overtax his digestive system. He had been accustomed to eating only once or twice a day with his junk snacks to provide the energy he was rapidly losing. With eating six small nutritionally balanced meals a day, he improved dramatically. His hypoglycemia was kept in check. Due to the nature of his job, numerous deadlines had to be met. At his clinical evaluation it was found that this generated a high level of stress which was adversely affecting his inadequate ability to maintain constant blood sugar levels. He was taught several different types of relaxation techniques to help him cope. Within one week after his initial visit his energy levels had begun to remain constant and within two weeks he had begun to remember those forgotten appointments, facts and figures. And his marriage? Still intact!

Asthma

Although the cause is unknown, it is believed to be a disease of the lungs with an environmental or ecological component. The present health care system emphasizes treatment of the symptoms, such as shortage of breath, often using steroids sucked from a bronchial dilator. But holistic doctors regard asthma as a chronic illness in which the need for medication could be reduced for many of the country's six million sufferers.

Asthmatics, holistic doctors have found, are often people with poor stress tolerance who unwittingly subject themselves to many allergies which trigger their attacks. These allergies can be due to air-polluting chemicals, grass, trees, certain foods, fungi, house dust or pollen, which irritate the lungs and then the nervous system, causing panic when breathing becomes difficult. That difficulty is not a blockage but a constriction through muscle spasm in the air tubes, causing labored breathing (as the word *asthma* means in Greek).

Having diagnosed the problem, the next step is to locate the allergy or allergies that trigger the spasms. With elimination of allergies, stress management and proper nutrition, asthmatics often learn to reduce the need for medication.

Ulcers

In the stomach or the intestinal system, ulcers are a weakness in the containing wall. That weakness is a small cavity or disintegration of the tissue. When this is irritated by stomach acids which digest food after a meal, it causes pain, nausea, vomiting and even bleeding in more serious cases. The pain can be, and often is, eased by taking an antacid tablet to neutralize the acid. But that does little for the underlying problem.

The problem can be resolved by letting the body heal its own ulcer—by reversing the process that caused it in the first place. This is done by changing the diet and by relaxation training. This is the method holistic doctors prefer. An operation might remove the ulcer, but will it stop the patient from getting another one? It is doubtful, because apart from his stressful life, the ulcer sufferer will probably keep on eating

the spicy foods and drinking coffee, tea and soda which—
along with his tobacco—are helping to irritate the ulcer.

Ulcerative Colitis

A chronic inflammation of the colon, the part of the intestine
that stores waste before it is expelled during bowel movements, colitis affects more women than men, usually after the
age of thirty. The initial symptoms (though it is very often
difficult for a doctor to determine the onset of the disease) are
feelings of weakness and tiredness, vague abdominal discomfort, and a slight change in frequency and consistency of the
stools. In its later stages it is more definite and patients experience cramps, lower abdominal pains and rectal bleeding.
The damage inside is similar to the stomach ulcer. The one-
sixteenth-inch-thick wall of the colon develops inflamed spots
and is irritated by movement, as it is either relaxed or filled
with stool. Holistic doctors have found that certain foods will
aggravate the symptoms and that altering the diet, moving
patients away from foods to which they may have
gastrointestinal allergies, has brought excellent results.

Headaches and Allergies

These words cover a broad spectrum of chronic illnesses that
are much more common and less vague than many people
imagine. To begin with, headaches do not "just happen;"
they can be symptoms of many different disorders. Some
headaches result from an allergic reaction to food, drink or
air pollution. The point is, they are not always the result of
emotional stress, or even eyestrain.

   Migraine is one of the worst types of chronic headaches.
British research shows that probably as many as 80 percent
of migraines are caused by an allergic reation to milk, chocolate, wheat, cheese, pork, wine or beer. As an example,

cheese, wine and beer all contain a chemical called tyramine which, when given to patients in its pure form during the British Migraine Association study, caused 40 out of 49 patients to have a migraine.

If the headache is *not* due to an organic cause, such as an allergy (which can be treated by removing the offending agent) or a brain tumor, it is likely to have a psychological cause. In that case, holistic doctors prefer to teach proper stress management, as opposed to prescribing Valium or Librium.

Apart from headaches, allergies show up as irregular heart rate, swelling of the feet, fatigue, runny nose, skin rashes, sickness and even epilepsy. They are caused by such simple substances as milk, soybean, beef, yeast, and wheat, along with complex chemicals such as phenol, chlorine and the hydrocarbons in the air.

Depression

While not quite as obvious a chronic illness, for many people it is a response to change or loss which happens, for instance, when there is a death in the family. This kind of depression goes away in time. But depression can also become chronic. Like headaches and other allergic reactions, it may *not* be psychological in origin. Very often there is a dietary reason; we have scientific proof that certain chemicals used as food additives cause depression. Yet many doctors will readily prescribe a mood-elevating drug to alleviate depression. One of the most widely used is Elavil, which holistic doctors believe serves only to suppress the symptoms.

Hypoglycemia can also cause depression, and holistic physicians have found that once these patients have reduced the sugar in their diet, they no longer get depressed without reason. The right diet provides the brain with sufficient energy and personality changes such as depression no longer occur.

From the holistic casebook:

Ted, a 57-year-old stonemason, showed symptoms of severe depression when he arrived at the
clinic in December—the time of year when many people feel depressed due to the holiday season approaching. We initially felt his depression was due to
this. However, upon further investigation we soon
learned he had been suffering in this way for some
eight years. He stated he had sought many types of
professional help ranging from hypnotists to conventional psychiatrists. He also complained of a chronically congested nose which later proved to be significant. As diagnosis progressed, it became apparent
that certain foods caused a change in his tempera-
ment as well as a worsening in his nasal congestion. A
series of allergy tests were suggested and these subsequently displayed many foods and environmental
sensitivities. Among them were products that had
been on a plate in front of him—soy and wheat. Now,
with the solution in hand came the task of teaching the
patient how to rotate those foods to which he had a
sensitivity. A series of consultations took place with
his wife present, and various tests were recommended. (We felt it important to bring his wife in on
the schedule so that she could support him in his new
dietary program.) This was particularly important as he
felt, quite strongly, that he had been eating what might
be a correct diet, i.e., mostly vegetables and whole
wheat bread. But both the wheat and the large
amounts of soy were disturbing his neurological system and once these were cut down he began to improve dramatically. And the significance of the nose?
Very few doctors would link allergies with depression
and this is why his blocked nose—a frequent "red
flag" in the field of food and environmental sensitivi-

ties—proved important. After three weeks of his new diet his nose cleared up too, and he was able to breathe freely through both nostrils.

Insomnia

One of the underlying causes of insomnia is stress, and it is far more successful to create a new lifestyle for the patient than to build him a drug habit he does not need. Many people who have difficulty sleeping at night are also depressed. Yet millions of Americans, instead of looking to stress reduction and dietary factors such as excess coffee and tea, endure a life of sleeping medication in order to get the rest their body needs.

From the holistic casebook:

Peter, a 45-year-old shoe salesman, had gone through more than two years of showing up for work with red eyes, slovenly appearance and constant fatigue. His friends and associates thought the years were just taking their toll. In fact, it was the nights, because he was suffering from chronic insomnia, one of the major health problems in the U.S. Many nights he would sleep, at the most, two to three hours, spending the remainder sitting in a chair in the dark, smoking cigarettes and trying to relax. He had tried many different treatments over the years ranging from a warm glass of milk to potent sleeping pills. The pills had been effective, but due to the ease of becoming addicted to them, he had tried to remedy his problem without their help. He came to the holistic clinic desperate for something different. He was given a thorough psychological examination as well as being questioned as

to his dietary and exercise habits. It was learned that
he was sedentary most of the time, only standing and
squatting occasionally to help his customers try on
their shoes. He also thought himself a failure in view
of the fact that his two older brothers were successful
businessmen. His meals consisted of grabbing fast
food from a nearby hamburger stand and he was taking no vitamin or mineral supplementation which
would be vital, considering his poor diet. A nutritional
evaluation was performed and it showed Peter to be
sadly lacking in a correct carbohydrate, protein and fat
ratio; these deficits were corrected by placing him on a
proper food program and a vitamin/mineral schedule.
He was also placed on an exercise program consisting
of jogging and swimming. He simultaneously worked
with a counselor in regard to his inferiority complex.
And the result? Within three months his problems began to ease and after a year of his new lifestyle he both
looked and acted like a totally different person.

Cirrhosis of the Liver

A chronic disease that often affects people who drink heavily,
cirrhosis is a fatty infiltration of the liver caused by the excessive alcohol, combined with poor eating habits. Unfortunately, most people do not know they have it until it is too late.
The first symptoms are nausea, gastrointestinal disturbances,
a change in the color of the stools, tiredness, weakness, and
sometimes darker urine. Many people often feel bloated as
fluid starts to accumulate because the liver, which detoxifies
the body, becomes overworked and loses ground with the intake of alcohol.

Holistic therapy can help control cirrhosis by giving the
patient high doses of B vitamins to support the liver and by
educating the patient in a new, alcohol-free lifestyle.

Alcoholism and Drug Addiction

The former is often the precursor of cirrhosis if a person drinks to reduce stress. Both seem to be related to complex hereditary and psychosocial problems, though the exact causes are not known. Most people have some knowledge of the social problems alcoholism and drug addiction create, and it would serve little purpose to illustrate the heartbreaking situations to which they lead.

Under the present medical care system, most heroin addicts, if they do eventually go for treatment, are merely transferred from one addictive drug to another (methadone) which is less harmful to their bodies. Holistic doctors, on the other hand, have successfully treated severe cases of drug addiction with high doses of vitamin C, stress reduction, exercise and better nutrition, creating a more natural lifestyle for the patient

Chronic Bronchitis

A respiratory disease affecting some six and one-half million Americans, bronchitis is more common among elderly people who may have worked in dusty occupations like factories or mines, had their homes in polluted areas, or—most significantly—smoked a lot of cigarettes. Sufferers have a chronic cough to get rid of mucus formation in the bronchial tubes.

From a holistic health point of view, chronic bronchitis is very much a preventable disease. That is because the coughing is caused when an irritant like cigarette smoke enters the lungs. The mucus forms to soothe the irritation, and in many people the cough can last for decades. The coughing is usually worse in the morning because the mucus has accumulated throughout the night.

Again, it is an illness that many people learn to live with, but education in the dangers of cigarette smoking, elimination of dusty atmospheres or pollution can reduce it to a

minor disorder. Chronic bronchitis in a nonsmoker is unusual, and if dust or pollution can be ruled out as the cause,
then allergic reations similar to those causing asthma are investigated.

Psoriasis

Psoriasis manifests itself as a skin rash anywhere on the body.
Those of you with shiny, scaly, itchy lesions on the knees,
legs, elbows or scalp should be checked for this chronic skin
disease. Stress and occasionally allergies seem to be aggravat-
ing factors in many patients.

Doctors ordinarily will treat psoriasis with steroids to
control the symptoms. Holistic physicians prefer to seek out
contributing factors, such as certain foods in the diet, and to
reduce the patient's stress response. Using this method, holistic doctors have achieved great success in keeping the problem under control while limiting the need for steroids.

Dandruff

A well-known complaint that is probably not thought of as a
chronic illness because it rarely causes any pain. But it is a
considerable discomfort to sufferers and, apart from being a
personal annoyance, often proves embarrassing in public
when your best friend is always the one to notice those white
specks on your shoulders.

What is happening is that the skin on your scalp flakes
off every time you brush or comb your hair. Treatment for
most people is with dandruff shampoo, which may suppress
it for a while. Holistic doctors prefer to deal with it from
within and have found definite improvements when stress,
which appears to make it worse, is reduced. Diet also seems
to be a large factor and when certain nutrients are increased,
dandruff can often be kept under control.

Acne

Another chronic disease that, like dandruff, is socially unacceptable. It particularly affects teenagers and in many cases, as parents will know, can be a source of considerable emotional trouble.

In severity it ranges from a few pimples to angry eruptions that can cause permanent scarring. Most people treat it with creams and lotions that are available without a prescription.

The inflammations occur because the skin's pores, which are outlets for the sweat glands, become plugged with a waxy substance called *sebum*. It is not fully understood just why that happens, but hormonal changes play some part in it.

In the holistic clinics, treatment of acne is usually centered on diet changes, use of zinc supplements and administering vitamin A, found in foods like carrots, eggs and green, leafy vegetables. That, of course, has to be coupled with cleanliness and meticulous skin care.

Sinusitis

A chronic infection of the sinuses, the passageways that arch from the top of the nose down to the windpipe. There are more than twenty million sufferers in the United States who get constant headaches and runny noses. The nasal passageways which are meant for inhaling are constantly blocked, so a dry mouth occurs from both inhaling and exhaling.

Many people endure it for decades and sniffle through life with decongestants and a funny voice. We have found the cause is often hydrocarbons from polluted air, or sometimes an allergy to a certain food. Once these have been cleared up, a nonsmoker can usually bring the condition down to a more tolerable level.

Diverticulosis and Diverticulitis

You have probably never heard of it, yet diverticulosis is the most common bowel disease in older people. It occurs in people who have chronic constipation.

The typical Western diet, high in fat and refined foods, takes between fifty and seventy hours to travel through your system. Not only are impurities longer in the system, but stools are smaller and much harder to expel, and are sometimes painful in severe cases.

A high-fiber diet composed of fruits, vegetables and cereals low in fat has a much shorter passage—some thirty hours—and less contact with the wall of the colon. Thus, sufferers of diverticulosis are advised to make a switch to a high-fiber diet to prevent diverticulitis (inflammation).

In a high-fat diet, stools are delayed in the large bowel, putting pressure on the very sensitive walls. This produces a pouch effect, or diverticulum. These become impacted and inflamed, bringing pain and sometimes fever, which then has to be treated as a crisis illness. A much better way to treat it, we believe, is with this switch to a bulkier, fibrous and fat-free diet, allowing a more natural remedy from within the body.

Tooth Decay

You might think tooth decay is the province of a dentist, not a doctor. You're right—if tooth decay to you means a filling, or worse, an extraction. But think again and you will see it really is a chronic illness—the filling is only the crisis point, as is the visit to the doctor when your arthritis flares up so badly you can no longer tolerate it.

Tooth decay begins before you even get an ache, with bacteria eating away at teeth you think you are taking care of by brushing twice daily. Unfortunately, the bacteria work on regardless, leeching minerals from your teeth until the gums are affected and you join the millions of American who have pyorrhea. More often than not, need we mention, you end up with a gleaming set of dentures.

Back then to the wily bacteria inside your mouth, proliferating daily on foods such as sugar, soda pop, and, surprisingly, high-protein foods like beefsteak. The holistic doctor's advice is: "Don't do them any favors." Eat fruits and vegetables, and proteins like cottage cheese which is high in calcium (just the mineral to strengthen the teeth), and you will starve those bacteria out. Couple that with good tooth care, not only brushing but flossing to free trapped food particles, and get set for a dramatic improvement.

Cancer

Current thinking of HEW Secretary Joseph Califano, supported by studies, indicates that a significant percentage of cancer will be environmentally or occupationally induced in the next generation. Despite limited funds being spent on prevention as opposed to cure, this seems to be the only solution for this chronic disease at present. Survival rates today are essentially no better than thirty years ago. Despite this, California law limits treatment to the so-called conventional therapies such as radiation, surgery and chemotherapy. The use of new therapies without the risk of criminal prosecution for doctors is pending in the courts at this time.

However, there are warning signs for cancer which you should be aware of, and though mostly they will prove to be false alarms, a visit to your physician may assist in the vital early detection of the disease. The American Cancer Society urges that every person "listen to their body" so that the following lifesaving signals do not go unheeded:

Symptom	*May indicate cancer of*
Change in bowel or bladder habits	Bowel or prostate
A sore that does not heal	Mouth or skin

Unusual bleeding or discharge	Uterus or bowel
Thickening or lump in breast (or elsewhere)	Breast (or other)
Indigestion or difficulty in swallowing	Stomach or esophagus
Obvious change in wart or mole	Skin
Nagging cough or hoarseness	Lung or larynx

A PILL FOR EVERY ILL?

The widespread use of man-made drugs to fight disease is relatively new in the field of medicine. In the early 1940s the idea of a pill for every ill became a popular notion, and today it has a firm footing in the minds of both doctor and patient. But if you are ill, using drugs to fight chronic disease is not something that should be taken lightly. There are many things that can go wrong and need to be considered before anyone embarks upon a course of therapy, and this is why holistic doctors are motivated towards using more natural healing processes. Drugs, in fact, are used as only a very last resort when all other weapons to fight chronic illness have failed.

Among physicians there is no doubt that wholesale over-prescribing is going on. In 1977, 60 million prescriptions were written for Valium alone, while in 1975 doctors made out a staggering 229 million prescriptions for mood-elevating drugs. What's more, adverse drug reaction is the seventh leading cause of hospitalization in the U.S.—and the treatment is costing the medical care system a whopping $3 billion annually. That is not to mention the cost in personal pain and suffering of those patients it affects. What's needed, says Donald Kennedy, commissioner of the FDA, is "sweeping overhaul such as happens only every quarter-century or so."

"We seem to have a belief that there is a drug for every

affliction . . . in which no visit to a physician is complete without ending in a written prescription," he told a 1978 convention of the Consumer Federation of America.

Much of the problem is the pressure applied to doctors by drug companies promoting their products. It begins in medical schools, where students get such offerings as stethoscopes and leather bags donated by the companies. In fact, the Association of American Medical Colleges say as much as $3500 per doctor per year is spent by the drug companies to peddle their products . . . a total of $1.4 billion across the country. And medical accessories are not the only "freebies." TV sets, tape recorders and other expensive items are handed out by salesmen to encourage doctors to prescribe their companies' drugs. Little wonder that bottle of pills makes a hole in your purse every time you visit the pharmacy.

One way to illustrate the problem would be to carry out a partial diagnosis of our fictitious character of the opening chapters and look at some of the drugs that might be prescribed for him if he were to visit his physician. Among his problems were gastritis (stomach upsets) and obesity. To counter those he *could* be prescribed at least two drugs: Librax (a combination of Librium to relieve anxiety and Quarzan to reduce stomach acid) for his gastritis and Fastin (an appetite depressant) to help reduce his weight.

Let us now look at just those two more closely, bearing in mind that for some people they seem to serve a purpose. For most, however, there are many potential dangers which you are entitled to, and should, know.

At the outset, Librax is classified by the FDA as being only "possibly" effective in the treatment of duodenal ulcers, so the odds on it achieving medical "miracles" seem slim. But more important, its general use, as with most drugs, is so fraught with dangers that physicians have to be given lengthy information about who not to prescribe it for, what can happen if it is prescribed, what precautions to take, and adverse reactions noted in pre-FDA classification tests. Here are some of them:

Librax contraindications: Should not be given to patients with glaucoma, enlarged prostate, benign bladder neck obstruction.

Librax warnings: (Physician should) caution patient about possible combined effects with alcohol, and against hazardous occupations requiring complete mental alertness, for example, operating machinery or driving.

Librax precautions: In the elderly and debilitated, dose must be limited to smallest effective amount to preclude ataxia (muscle incoordination), over-sedation and confusion.

Librax adverse reactions: Syncope (fainting), skin eruptions, minor menstrual irregularities, nausea, constipation, dryness of mouth, blurring of vision, urinary hesitancy.

Fastin, an amphetamine-related drug, has just as many risk factors, yet the manufacturer, in typical medical journal advertisements, coaxes the physician to prescribe it to this patient with all the flair that Madison Avenue can offer.

"Use Fastin to fill in all the emptiness of hunger during the failure-prone beginning weeks of his diet," urges the blurb after setting up a cozy doctor-patient drama that sees the best-laid plans to diet blown away by the "hollow call of hunger." As it may, but is it worth it, when you know this . . .?

Fastin contraindications: Should not be given to patient with advanced arteriosclerosis, symptomatic cardiovascular disease, moderate to severe hypertension.

Fastin warnings: Tolerance develops within a few weeks, rendering the drug ineffective, not to mention the abuse potential among drug addicts.

Fastin precautions: Physicians are warned to use caution in prescribing the drug to anyone with even mild hypertension.

Fastin adverse reactions: Palpitation, elevation of blood pressure, restlessness, dizziness, insomnia, constipation, headache, impotence.

From the holistic casebook:

George, a 56-year-old mechanic working two jobs to make ends meet, presented himself to the HMG clinic with increasingly severe headaches. He was 30 lbs. overweight and had a history of high blood pressure, which was out of control—partly because of his dislike of taking medication on a regular basis. Thorough medical examination by a previous physician had revealed no underlying cause for his high blood pressure, and he was told to cut down on his salt intake and use the medication he so disliked.* It was obvious that this patient would need something more radical if he was to show improvement. More detailed history upon his HMG evaluation revealed that he was under tremendous stress, calming his nerves by drinking some twelve cups of coffee daily and biting his fingernails. After confirming the previous physician's diagnosis, George was placed on a very specific low-salt, low-calorie diet and given nutritional counseling in the foods to eat and to avoid. He was enrolled in a program of stress management and placed on an exercise regime after physiological examination of his cardiovascular system by treadmill exercise testing. Inside 60 days he was 30 lbs. lighter and asymptomatic.

Clearly, drugs are not the answer to today's health care problems. The manufacturers, however, remain undaunted.

"The pharmaceutical industry spends more money on the advertising and promotion of prescription drugs than

---

*The patient's medications included Aldomet, Hydrodiuril, and Reserpine, all of which are designed to lower blood pressure. They controlled his symptoms, but as is common in many similar patients, the side effects of impotence and depression influenced his decision to abandon them for a more natural method.

they do on research into the development of new products,"
Senator Edward Kennedy disclosed during a Senate investigation into the entire drug manufacturing field of medicine.

More surgery does not appear to be the answer either. In
fact, there is so much top-level concern about excessive surgery being carried out in hospitals across the country that the
Department of Health, Education and Welfare is officially
advising all patients to seek a second opinion before going
under the knife. The move was largely based on a 1976 report by the House Subcommittee on Oversight and Investiga-
tions that claimed that 2.38 million operations were performed unnecessarily in 1974.

That was 17 percent of all operations and cost the public
$4 billion as well as, estimates the American College of Sur-
geons, 11,900 lives. Furthermore, the report revealed:

• Studies in Kansas, Vermont and Maine found a direct
correlation between the higher rates of surgery and the number of surgeons and facilities.

• The overall rate of surgery was 31 percent higher in
the Midwest than the South.

• The overall rate of surgery in the United States increased by 23 percent between 1970 and 1975—and even
now the same surgery rate is growing four times faster than
the population.

In a separate study presented at the American Public
Health Association meeting in Los Angeles in 1978, there
was new evidence to suggest surgery actually kills a significant number of people. In Los Angeles County in 1976, during a five-week-long doctors' slowdown, the death rate
dropped sharply when surgery was reduced by 58 percent,
compared with a similar period in 1975.

Before we move away from the subject of surgery, it
should perhaps be noted that an estimated $1 billion could be
saved just be eliminating overnight hospital stays for women
undergoing minor gynecological surgery.

Not many procedures escape overutilization, even when
dangerous radiation is involved. A 1978 government report

questioned the value of routine X-rays, in hospitals, for head injuries. As a test, a group of Seattle physicians reduced them by 40 percent; it was found that this did not affect the accuracy of the overall diagnosis. In other words, many physicians needlessly expose patients to unnecessary radiation instead of looking for signs and symptoms of injury, which during a careful examination can be accurately read.

Obviously, this ludicrous system must gradually be brought under control and solutions looked for in the prevention of illness and disease. It is no longer feasible to have a system which waits for people to get into a crisis and then tries to find an answer. We must, as some government officials appear to recognize, switch the accent from disease to health. This is what holistic physicians have created by looking at the patient as a total human being, considering his relationship to his environment, his lifestyle, his work, pleasure, and daily living habits. It is humanistic medicine, not a medicine that looks at organs and disease fighting each symptom on a one-to-one basis.

Holistic doctors are not theorizing about what might or might not happen with preventive processes. They have actually implemented a system that is the most economical and the most practical. Prevention is effective in the fight against disease. Obviously, if you eat one fast-food hamburger and drink a glass of soda pop you will not necessarily become ill. But there is enough evidence available today to show that if you eat a faulty diet over a period of time, you may develop a chronic degenerative disease. If you are unable to deal with life's stresses, not able to cope with your environment, then you are prone to illness.

Yet industry still has not recognized that there is a problem. The sugar processors are still saying that it does not hurt to overconsume their product. The dairy industries have averted controls that would curb overconsumption of their products. And one of the most powerful economic forces in the country, the tobacco industry, outspends the government's antismoking drive by ten to one in its research to de-

velop a so-called "safe" cigarette. Even in the medical
equipment industry, twice as much is spent annually to develop an artificial heart as is spent to prevent cardiovascular
disease.

Why is prevention such a dirty word? There are many
reasons:

• There is inadequate health education in the present
system. The nation has only one health educator in schools
and medical facilities for every 17,000 people—compared
with one *doctor* for every 515 people.

• Even though the nation's mortality statistics are dom-
inated by death from such diseases as cancer and heart problems—which are related to nutrition—the education of most
doctors includes little on the subject.

• Medical technology has ongoing capital and labor in-
vestments tied up in fighting disease. Physicians are continually being trained to use increasingly more complicated
equipment, and ultimately come to depend on it.

• There is a negative attitude on the part of the public.
Many people prefer to ignore prevention because to them it
means giving up something or being inconvenienced for a
promise of reward in years to come. There is also widespread
apathy because there is no personal motivation unless there is
sickness. Like our fictitious sick character, there is a "put
off" attitude because the illness is chronic rather than crit-
ical. Then, when the crisis comes, there is often an unrealistic
expectation about the ability of medicine to cure the disease.

• Medical insurance schemes may call themselves
"health" insurance, but they are in fact "disease" insurance.
Both private and government insurance schemes willingly
pay for diagnosis and treatment of disease, but not for prevention. Medicare excludes payment for preventive services
to the elderly and Medicaid pays only for periodic health
screening for children.

• There is a negative attitude among doctors. Prevention, to many, is intellectually dull. It is without challenge.
The approach to it seems banal and pedestrian when there is

the excitement and glamor of today's high-technology thera-
peutics. It is comparatively unexciting to change people's
lives, as holistic doctors do. Most physicians prefer to stay
locked in combat with the diseases of our times.

There is an economic aspect to that, too. Under the present health-care system, doctors get paid for disease-fighting
procedures, not for sitting and chatting with patients to help
them get into harmony with the world.

But if a doctor doesn't get excited by getting someone
well, then is he really being a doctor? Holistic physicians, like
any professional listener, acknowledge that this sort of counseling could be somewhat removed from the intellectual challenges of medicine. Many, as we have in the HMG, now use
ancillary support groups to spread the load so that each patient sees not only the doctor, but nurses and paramedical
staff specializing in each aspect of changing to a life of disease prevention.

People seem to be more and more willing to call on physicians for this kind of attention, because there is a massive
population, growing by the day, that needs, and increasingly
desires, to be educated in a new health care system. There is
no greater reward for a true doctor than to be told by his patient: "I never felt better in my life." And that is happening.

The question really is "What is the goal of medicine?" Is
it for people to be healthy? Or is it for people to get sick and
then find some way to cure them? The American way at the
moment is the latter. Holistic doctors prefer to try to achieve
in all people what the World Health Organization defines as
health: "A state of *complete* physical, mental, and social
well-being."

Goodbye to the Old: Ring in the New

You probably think that heart attack or a "crippling" bout of arthritis will never happen to you. But if you have experienced even mild chronic illness, the degeneration in your body has already started. The choice you have to make now is "Do I genuinely want to stop it?" There is no need for decline. Going downhill is not as inevitable a part of growing old as you might think. Your body will not stay young forever, but degeneration can be dramatically slowed. But remember, the Feeling Good Scale is only a rough indicator of your present level of well-being. Now is the time to be much more exact about your health, and this is done by formulating a more accurate appraisal of how you are coping with life.

The following questions might seem unusual. They might possibly be questions about your life that you never really answered before. But they are important and should be noted, for your body does not go through life without registering the insults. Everything takes its toll—the worthless food, the chemicals in the air, the stress, the lack of exer-

cise—all may be precursors to illness. Study each question
carefully and mark the ones which are relevant with a "yes."
Then look at them again, and by turning the questions into
direct statements you will have part of the picture of you as
you are now, and you will be in a position to investigate what
is happening to you.

1. Are you really unhappy or discontented for any reason?
2. Have you been feeling unusually depressed or discouraged lately?
3. Do you consider yourself nervous?
4. Have you any special problem constantly on your mind?
5. Do you often feel tense and keyed up so that you have trouble falling asleep at night?
6. Do you think you need more sleep than you are getting?
7. Do you have one or more drinks of liquor per day?
8. Are you concerned about your drinking?
9. Are you anxious to change your occupation for any reason?
10. Are you working too hard?
11. Would you rather be doing something else than work?
12. Do you have trouble getting along with co-workers?
13. Do you disagree often with your boss?
14. Do you cry easily?
15. Is your home life unpleasant?
16. Do you have uncontrollable flares of anger?
17. Do you bite your fingernails?
18. Are you extremely shy or sensitive?
19. Does every little thing get on your nerves?
20. Are you the worrying type?

A questionnaire similar to this is given to patients on their
first visit to the HMG clinics. The results do not by any

means complete the picture. It is also important for a doctor
to know what drugs a patient is taking. Drugs cause artificial
reactions in the body and, as you already know, one of the
main aims of holistic health is to separate patients and drugs
altogether. See if any of these apply to you.

Ask yourself if you ever take: Laxatives, sedatives,
tranquilizers, sleeping pills, aspirin, stomach antacids, hormones, steroids, thyroid medication, appetite depressants,
pep pills, nitroglycerine, diuretics, water pills, antibiotics,
anticoagulants (blood thinners), antihistamines (cold tablets),
insulin for diabetes, heart medication (digitalis), blood pressure medication, or kidney disease medication.

More than likely, when you review your answers, you
will have given yourself something of a shock. If you are an
average person, you will have a whole arsenal of those drugs
in your medicine cabinet ready for that upset stomach or
headache. Reaching for them is almost a reflex action.

Apart from introducing insults into your body, it is cost-
ly if you add up what you spend in the drugstore every year.
The body has many of the healing mechanisms it needs if you
just know how to trigger them. As with chronic illnesses
themselves, home remedies become as much a habit as walking, talking, sleeping and eating. Television and other advertising pressures make it seem perfectly reasonable to get ill
and then dash out for a remedy. But these drugs are marketed
in the same way as cars or appliances. The manufacturers
purposely set out to create a psychological need and make
you feel that you must fulfill that need. The thought of being
without the crutch of a painkiller or a tranquilizer might fill
you with horror, but you really don't need them. Any holistic
patient would tell you that.

The next step in building your picture concentrates on
the actual condition of your body and the symptoms you
have at the present time. This is what we call "looking for the
warning signs." In many cases they are so subtle that you
have probably dismissed them as just part of the hazards of
living. It is, however, very important for you to know what

they are so you will ignore them no longer. When you look at the questions, you'll immediately recognize whether the symptom applies to you or not. Of course, there are no right or wrong answers. It is not a quiz to see how many points you can win, but simply to gain an insight into the degeneration that can take place in your body.

SKIN

Have you ever had:
1. A persistent rash on your skin?
2. A skin allergy or hives?
3. Infections or diseases of the skin?
4. Exposure to strong chemicals or poisons?
5. Problems with body odor?
6. Unusual loss of hair?
7. A sore that does not heal?
8. Unusual prolonged bleeding from cuts or wounds?
9. Really black (not dark brown) mole anywhere on your skin?
10. Any skin blemish increasing in size?

EYES

1. Do you wear glasses all or part of the time?
2. Do you have pain in or around your eyes?
3. Does pus or matter collect in your eyes frequently?
4. Do you have trouble with your distant or near vision?
5. Do you ever see double?
6. Do you have trouble distinguishing colors?
7. Do you occasionally see spots in front of your eyes?

8. Do you have difficulty seeing clearly at night?
9. Are there any blind spots in your vision?
10. Do you have difficulty seeing out of the corners of your eyes?

EARS

1. Are you having difficulty hearing?
2. Are you deaf in either ear?
3. Have you ever had a running ear?
4. Have you noticed buzzing or other noises in your ears?
5. Have you ever had your eardrums punctured?
6. Have you ever had earache or discharge from either ear?
7. Have you ever had bleeding from your ears?
8. Do you easily become sick from motion of car, train or ship?
9. Do you have frequent dizzy spells or lightheadedness?
10. Do you frequently lose your balance?

NOSE

1. Do you have frequent or severe nosebleeds?
2. Are you often bothered with a running nose?
3. Do you have postnasal drip (thick mucus in throat)?
4. Is your nose constantly stuffed up?
5. Do you have difficulty recognizing common odors?
6. Is part of your face swollen and painful when you have head colds (sinus trouble)?
7. Do you have severe headaches with head colds?

8. Have you ever had a nose injury?
9. Do you often catch colds?

MOUTH AND THROAT

1. Do you have a feeling of a choking lump in your throat?
2. Do you suffer from frequent bouts of swollen glands in your neck?
3. Have you noticed recurrent hoarseness or recent voice change?
4. Do you have frequent toothaches?
5. Do you see a dentist once a year?
6. Has your dentist any trouble stopping your bleeding after tooth extraction?
7. Do you wear dentures and do they fit well?
8. Have you any sores on lips or mouth that don't heal?
9. Are your gums or tongue frequently sore, sensitive or bleeding?
10. Have you ever had tonsilitis or quinsy?

CARDIOVASCULAR SYSTEM

1. Do you have a cough when you lie down?
2. Have you ever had high blood pressure, heart trouble or heart murmur?
3. Have you ever been awakened in the middle of the night with chest pains or shortness of breath, having to sit up to catch your breath?
4. Do you have chest pains when moving arms, bending, turning, coughing, lying down or deep breathing?
5. After climbing stairs or walking, do you have to stop because of chest pains or shortness of breath?

6. Have you ever had a severe chest pain behind the breastbone, radiating to shoulder, jaw, hand or abdomen?
7. Do you have severe chest pains after eating, belching, prolonged walking or emotional upset?
8. Does your heart often race or skip a beat?
9. Have you noticed any ankle swelling?
10. Do you have leg cramps when walking and/or resting?
11. In cold weather or in cold water do you have pain in your fingers or toes?

DIGESTIVE SYSTEM

1. Do you have trouble swallowing or does your food stick midway down?
2. Do you often have gnawing pains or a burning in the pit of your stomach between meals or in the middle of the night?
3. Does stomach distress keep you from eating certain foods (spicy or fried foods, coffee, alcohol)?
4. Have you ever vomited blood or bile, or passed black tarry stools?
5. Is stomach distress relieved by milk, food or bicarbonate?
6. Is it common for you to feel weak or break into a sweat a few hours after eating?
7. Do you often suffer from heartburn, indigestion or gas?
8. Do you eat in a hurry and at irregular times?
9. Are you constipated (two or more days without a bowel movement)?
10. Do you have piles (hemorrhoids) or bright red blood with your bowel movement?
11. Do you have frequent diarrhea?

URINARY TRACT

1. Have you ever had a kidney or bladder infection?
2. Have you ever had swelling or puffiness around your face or eyes?
3. Have you ever had sugar in your urine?
4. Have you ever passed blood in your urine?
5. Do you freqeuntly get up at night to urinate?
6. Have you felt any pain when urinating?
7. Have you ever had trouble starting or maintaining a strong force of urine stream?
8. Have you ever had trouble stopping urine stream (dribbling)?
9. Have you ever had difficulty in holding your urine?
10. Have you ever had back pains related to urinating?

MUSCLE SYSTEM

1. Did you have "growing pains" as a child?
2. Do you have pains moving from joint to joint, associated with fever and sore throat?
3. Do you have neck, upper or lower back pain made worse by moving and helped by rest?
4. Do you suffer from pains in your joints, muscles or bones?
5. Have you ever had swollen, red or stiff joints?
6. Have you ever been told you have bursitis, rheumatism or gout?
7. Do you have attacks of joint pains after exertion, eating or drinking too much?
8. When using your joints, do you have a rubbing or grating sensation?
9. Do you have joint pains or stiffness that are

worse in the morning and improve during the day?

10. Do you have back pain that travels into one or both of your legs?

NERVOUS SYSTEM

1. Do you have frequent headaches?
2. Do you have headaches associated with pain and pulsation of blood vessels in temples?
3. Do you have headaches associated with watery eyes or running nose?
4. Do you have headaches that wake you up out of a sound sleep and are constant in location?
5. Do you have dizziness when turning your head quickly?
6. Do you have dizziness associated with a whistling sound, nausea or difficulty in hearing?
7. Do you have headaches with tightness in your neck and scalp muscles or with the sensation of a tight band about your head?
8. Has any part of your body ever been paralyzed or always numb?
9. Have you been bothered by not being able to talk distinctly?
10. Have you had some impairment of your arms, legs or hands due to tremor or spasm?
11. Do you have a tingling feeling in your fingers or toes?

GLANDULAR SYSTEM

1. Do you have any persistent or recurring pains in any part of your body?

2. Are you unduly sensitive to heat or cold?
3. Have you had any thyroid trouble?
4. Have you had weight loss of more than 10 pounds in the last six months?
5. Have you had any weight increase of more than 10 pounds in the last year?
6. Has your weight stayed constant in the last five years?

BLOOD

1. Have you ever had a blood transfusion reaction?
2. Have you had any unexplained excessive weakness or fatigue of more than three weeks in duration?
3. Do you have varicose veins?
4. Have you, or did you have, phlebitis?
5. Do you have any swollen glands in neck, armpits, groin or elsewhere?
6. Do you have bleeding from any body opening?
7. Were you ever told you were anemic?

Isn't it remarkable how many things can go wrong? And yet these are only some of the most common symptoms of illness in the miracle that is the human body. Obviously it is not possible to glean a diagnosis from your answers unless you do it jointly with a physician; but for you as a reader, diagnosis is not the main objective. Just by being made conscious of all the problems that can cause upsets in the body and learning about their significance, you are already a better person than you were. You are wiser and more knowledgeable about yourself, and even if you could only find a handful of questions that related to you, you will be in a position now, if you so choose, to act and correct them with your physician's help.

The HMG moves at this point from the theoretical to the practical with all new patients, taking them through various diagnostic procedures. It is purposely a much broader based investigation than most ordinary doctors would undertake and there is a reason for that. It is that the holistic physician sees little value in dealing with isolated problems. It is far better in getting to the root of chronic illness to deal with everything at once, looking at various areas of the body to see if one aspect might be affecting the other. To do this the HMG has brought under one roof some of the finest and most sophisticated diagnostic aids available, and therefore patients get all the benefits of the old with the new.

These have been found extremely beneficial in helping doctors in early low-risk detection of disease. Holistic doctors strongly hope that more physicians will follow their lead in bringing such equipment and procedures from the hospitals and specialty clinics into everyday family practices. It is extremely important to emphasize that in the diagnostic evaluation of the patient, the testing procedures used have as low a risk as possible. In today's medical world, many potentially dangerous tests are performed because physicians do not carry out thorough histories and physical examination. Also, more dramatic procedures bring the doctor greater reimbursement. For example, with the increasing numbers of bypass surgeries performed, there has been a dramatic rise in the number of angiograms, (an invasive test in which dye is injected into the arteries to check circulation) carried out, which result in a death rate of approximately 1 percent.

One of the guiding principles of holistic doctors is, if you are not sure you can help your patient, at least do not hurt him. The point is: attempt nontoxic, noninvasive methods first.

Briefly, these are some of the noninvasive diagnostic tools that you can expect to find in many holistic clinics:

Thermography. Used to diagnose stroke potential, arteriosclerosis, any many other circulatory problems. It records the flow of blood through the body by recording skin temperature and producing a photographic color print.

Plethysmography. Similar to the electrocardiogram, it measures the blood flow through vessels in arms, legs, fingers, toes and head. It reveals the presence of hardening of the arteries at early stages.

Doppler Ultrasound. One of the newest diagnostic tools, ultrasound is a potential replacement for dangerous X-rays and is used in screening for circulatory diseases.

Stress Treadmill Electrocardiogram. The stress ECG is used as a guide for recommending a balanced exercise program in addition to detecting unsuspected heart disease. The heart rate is recorded while the person walks on an elevated treadmill.

Pulmonary Function Testing. Determines lung capacity by measuring the amount of air a person can blow in and out of the lungs.

Heidelberg Capsule. Permits the measurement of acid in the stomach and intestine by means of radio signals which allow the physician to analyze test results as the capsule travels through the patient's gastrointestinal tract. This eliminates the need for the unpleasant procedure of swallowing a stomach tube.

Mineral Analysis. A tissue and serum analysis is made for detection of trace minerals and metals. New evidence is being uncovered linking the excess of certain minerals such as lead and cadmium—and the lack of minerals such as zinc—with a variety of disorders including high blood pressure.

The diagnostic procedures to detect food and chemical allergies and hypoglycemia need to be discussed more fully. They are important because they are tests for chronic illnesses that are very much a sign of our times. Both cause a variety of symptoms and allergies and can be the cause of other chronic illnesses. Doctors in holistic medicine regard both these problems as a major part of their work because both are controllable, yet cause a myriad of undiagnosed pain and suffering for many.

The following is a quiz devised to help tell you whether you have hypoglycemia. Answer all the questions honestly, placing a mark either in the zero, monthly, weekly or daily column, before reading on.

Check the frequency with which you experience:

Zero   Monthly   Weekly   Daily

1. Inability to concentrate
2. Excessive fatigue
3. Nervousness and
   irritability
4. Depression.
5. Apprehensions.
6. Excessive weakness
7. Insomnia.
8. Headaches.
9. Dizziness and
   light-headedness.
10. Digestive disturbances.
11. Forgetfulness.
12. Indecisiveness.
13. Blurred vision.
14. Craving for sweets.
15. A need for alcohol.
16. Difficulty getting back to
    sleep if you awaken
    at night.
17. Heavy breathing.
18. Bad dreams.
19. Bleeding gums.
20. Brown spots or skin
    bronzing.
21. Easy bruising.

22. A need for coffee in the morning.
23. A need to work without pressure.
24. Nervous exhaustion.
25. Convulsions.
26. Crying for no reason.
27. Eating to calm nerves.
28. Faintness if meal is delayed.
29. Shakiness if hungry.
30. Hallucinations.
31. Hand tremors.
32. Exaggerated emotions.
33. Between-meals nibbling.
34. Lack of energy.
35. Moodiness and the blues.
36. Sleepiness after eating.

Totals:

To find your score give yourself three points for each symptom you checked in the daily column, two points in the weekly column, one point in the monthly column, and nothing for the zero column. Then add them up at the bottom of the list and calculate your total score.

If you are healthy and able to utilize all the carbohydrates you eat and drink, your score should be 30 or less. Indeed, holistic doctors contend that a truly healthy person would get a score of 0–15. If you scored in the 30–70 range, there is a good reason for suspicion that you already have early signs of hypoglycemia. Above that figure, you are probably affected and may even have an allergy to sugar as the cause of the symptoms. A glucose tolerance test and allergy testing would confirm any findings.

Food and Chemical Allergies.

An allergic reaction can often come about by consuming too
much of a certain sensitive food. Finding that sensitivity is
not as simple as it may sound. Everybody consumes so many
different types of foods and chemicals and breathes in so
many different types of chemicals and pollution, that it can
be a painstaking job finding which one, or ones, are causing
the insult to the body. To help, the HMG uses the *provocative*
or *sublingual* testing system. Both terms refer to provoking a
reaction from the patient by placing the suspected substance
on the mucous membrane under the tongue, where it is immediately absorbed.

We have found that well over half the people tested in
our clinics have ecological sensitivities. Indeed, enough for us
to need extra qualified staff to carry out the testing. This, of
course, is done under the complete supervision of the doctor
and he is advised after every stage. For successful testing, the
patient has to prepare by not eating for a few hours prior to
testing. This is necessary to keep the body clear of other foods
which might disguise the reaction, making it simpler to isolate the troublemaker. Also, because outside or environmental insults might be responsible, the part of the clinic where
the testing is done is kept as clear as possible, without in-
terference from cigarette smoke, perfumes and other
cosmetics, and outside pollutants. In a natural atmosphere,
the testing begins.

It is a procedure that will amaze you. Simply by dropping under your tongue an extract of a food you might enjoy
or of a chemical from the air, an instant reaction of dizziness,
fatigue, nervousness, muscle and joint pain or headache may
be brought on. Then, as quickly as it is induced, it can be
stopped by dropping a neutralizing dosage onto the very
same mucous membrane. The results are quite convincing to
our patients when we are able to turn the reactions on and off
at will. We have even demonstrated that certain foods can
cause some people to fall asleep, and we've been able to wak-

en them by neutralizing the reaction. If we find that there is a food which brings a reaction in our patient (and the foods are as common as corn, milk or beef), they are then shown how to test themselves with everything that they eat. It is a case of deliberately eating only one food per meal and waiting for the symptoms to occur and then adjusting the diet accordingly.

After a while, it will be found which foods are "good" and which are "bad," but this does not mean the "bad" foods have to be avoided completely. You may have to abstain for a while to allow the body to recover after years of headaches, say, from milk allergy. These foods can then be reintroduced in a limited way by eating or drinking the troublesome food only once or twice a week instead of several times daily. In many cases, nutrients and vitamins can be preescribed to help the body's natural defenses against allergic substances.

Reactions to chemicals are a slightly different matter, but it is possible to isolate roughly where the problem may lie by looking closely at your own living and working conditions. The pollutant you are being exposed to may well be removable, or conversely, you could avoid it by a simple change in habits. If necessary, a vaccination against the offending agent can be prepared. The following questionnaire will give you some idea what we mean about pollutants in your environment.

Your Environmental History

Check as applicable.

Home

How long have you lived there?
Single house
Double house
Apartment
Hotel or dormitory
Trailer

Region

City residential
City industrial
Suburban
Small town
Rural

Garage

In separate unattached building
With inside passageway between house and garage
In basement of house
None

Occupation

Distance between home and work

Work Region

City
Suburban
Small town
Rural

Travel to Work by

Car
Bus
Train
Walking
Other

Heating and Ventilation of Home

Fuel   *Type*

Gas   Warm air

Oil
Electric
Coal
Other

Hot water or steam
Electric—heat pump or
   radiant (circle which)
Space heaters
Fireplaces

Air Conditioning

Window units
Central system
Filters—fiberglass
   oiled
   unoiled
   electrostatic
   activated
   carbon
Automobile—factory installed
         installed after
         car purchase

Kitchen Exhaust

Fan—yes
    no
Kitchen door—usually
        open
Kitchen door—usually
        closed

Utilities

Range

Age of unit
electric
gas
oil

Refrigerator

Age of unit
electric
gas

Clothes Dryer

Age of unit
Gas

Water Heater

Electric
Gas

Food Storage

In glass
In plastic
In enamel ware
In aluminium foil

Drinking Water

Spring or well
Softened
Chlorinated
Fluoridated

If you discover, in filling out the questionnaire, that you have a substantial exposure to gas appliances, it would be wise to have them checked for proper functioning and to install new filters. By process of elimination, try to find out which aspect of your life is causing you problems. We recommend as little gas in the house as possible; it's likely that the blocked sinuses that have bothered you for years might well have been caused by the dry, polluted air that gas creates.

It is best to check with a doctor if you suspect you are a victim of your environment, rather than enduring allergic reactions for years to come. As a general guide, it is wise to seek as clean an atmosphere as possible in which to live and work, and also reduce your exposure to city air and other pollutants as much as you can.

For food storage, it is advisable to change to glass containers, as plastic, enamel and aluminum have the potential to give off chemicals harmful to the body.

Drinking of tap water should be avoided. We doubt that many traditional doctors would take us to task over this assertion. In many rural districts the water may be pure and natural, but it is accepted that in practically every city in the United States the tap water is polluted. This is due not only to the generally dirty environment, but to purifying agents, which over the long term can produce side effects such as headaches and stomach upsets. The harmful effects of drinking tap water do not appear suddenly; it has to be consumed over a long period of time for the effects to be evident. We strongly advise all our patients to change permanently to bottled spring water, which is not expensive, can be delivered to your home, and is refreshing and full of minerals good for the body. We have discovered during testing that apart from the high levels of toxic metals in polluted tap water, high levels of copper and lead are being absorbed into the body from the pipes the water has come through.

From the holistic casebook:

Edna is a 30-year-old housewife who came to the clinic complaining of a history of ulcerative colitis. She had been experiencing periods of severe abdominal cramping with blood in her stools. She had had the problem for the past six years and was progressively getting worse. During this time she had engaged several different categories of physicians ranging from general practitioners to gastrointestinal specialists. Their treatment had predominantly consisted of medication to control her symptoms. It had alleviated the problem for only brief periods of time. Finally, her last physician suggested surgery as a cure for her illness. She was advised to have part of her intestine, which had been affected by the disease, removed. In desperation she sought out a nonsurgical treatment. Upon her first examination and from personal history it was found that the patient had episodes of abdominal pain after eating certain foods. She consequently was put through a series of food allergy tests and was placed on a diet which bypassed those foods to which she had shown an adverse reaction. These included milk, milk products, soy and wheat, which had been irritating her intestinal tract and causing pain and bleeding. Upon following her new diet, Edna began to improve. It was also discovered that she was under some stress, apparently caused by her inability to engage in certain sports she had loved as a younger woman. This exacerbated her problem and a series of encounter groups helped her realize this and control her frustrations. This led to a further improvement of her condition. The patient was finally able to be taken off her medication. In a year and a half she had only two attacks of colitis which were far less severe than those she had previously experienced. To date, surgery is not even contemplated.

Willa, a 37-year-old mother of two teenage children, came to the clinic complaining of constant headaches, chronic fatigue and daily nasal congestion which gave her difficulty breathing. She had previously been treated by a neurologist for her headaches. That treatment had included doses of potent pain-killing drugs which she had to take just to be able to carry out her normal day-to-day activities. Her life had become unbearable, causing her to be totally dependent on her "lifesaving" pills. Diagnostic procedures included a glucose tolerance test, food and chemical allergy tests and a blood analysis. The patient was diagnosed to have low blood sugar, multiple allergies and clinical hypothyroidism. She was placed on a restrictive diet with specific mineral and vitamin supplementation. She was also given a slight amount of natural thyroid medication and environmental adjustments were made. The patient initially felt worse with her new nutritional program. This worsening state continued for a period of approximately two weeks, at which time she began to experience less severe headaches. This improvement in the degree of pain continued until finally she was symptom free without the use of her medication. This was achieved within six weeks from the onset of her treatment. Her energy simultaneously increased as well as almost a permanent resolving of her nasal congestion. This was brought about by the removal of various offending agents in her environment, including plastics and chlorine, which had been irritating the mucous membranes in her sinus passages.

The problem of toxic absorption leads to the first treatment prescribed for HMG patients—cleansing the body of potentially harmful chemicals and foods. This is done with a "detoxification fast," which is like a spring cleaning for the

body and is beneficial because it acts as a firm foundation for
the new lifestyle.

The fast we recommend for most HMG clinic patients al-
lows the overworked gastrointestinal system of the body to
take a well-deserved rest. It also has a very important effect
on the actual cells, allowing old ones to be destroyed and new
ones to form in a process known as *auto-digestion.*This is
beneficial because many of the cells destroyed are fat cells.
Considerable weight loss can be enjoyed.

The fast should be seen not only as a benefit for the body,
but also for the mind. If it is approached wholeheartedly in
this way there will be no discomfort whatsoever. In fact,
once the hunger pangs of the first couple of days are over-
come—and perhaps a little dizziness which is a normal with-
drawal reaction—you will have surprisingly more energy
than you have had for a long time.

During this time, you will not be completely without
food. For most people, total abstention from food can be
traumatic. We recommend that they consume watermelon,
which is a completely fat-free food and so simple to digest
that it does not affect the resting of the gastrointestinal system. Along with the melon, spring water needs to be drunk
regularly to flush out the system. As the two go on their way
through your body, it is easy to imagine them drawing out
the poisons and chemicals that have built up in your body
over the years.

Some patients, we have found, are not strong enough to
withstand a four- to seven-day fast of this nature or it is not
indicated because of their medical condition. For them we
prescribe a special vegetable broth consisting of sufficient
nutrients to help them endure the week of not eating regular
meals. This is not as good as the watermelon fast, but many
of the benefits are still obtained. At the end of the fast, normal food intake is resumed gradually, to allow the body to
begin its digestive duties once again. We do not recommend
that anyone fast unless they are under the supervision of a
physician.

From the holistic casebook:

Zena, a 54-year-old music teacher, had been ill for several months with fatigue, aching muscles and joints. Her condition, she complained, had been worsening rapidly. Her livelihood was teaching young students how to play the piano and this she was finding progressively more difficult; she was contemplating giving up her profession. She preferred a holistic clinic because of the natural methods of treatment it offered. Upon diagnosis it was discovered that she had rapidly progressing arthritis which was seriously affecting the movement of her joints, not the least of them her fingers on the keyboard. After the appropriate evaluation she was placed on a detoxification fast which dramatically increased her energy. (Before coming to the clinic, Zena had been attempting to establish a vitamin and mineral schedule on her own. Dosages, however, had been erratic due to her being influenced by a multitude of differing, yet "authoritative" opinions. Needless to say, the supplementations had been of little value to her condition.) After reviewing the results of her comprehensive testing, a stable vitamin and mineral schedule was established, and she was presented with a series of exercises for her stiffening joints and within a few weeks managed to continue with only a minimal level of anti-inflammatory medication. She was once again to return to her piano and the life she loved.

Fasting is not indicated for people with severe cardiovascular disease, severe diabetes, or heavy metal toxicity, who would probably have placed themselves at around 40 percent on our Feeling Good Scale. For these, holistic medicine offers an alternative to any treatment they might have to undergo in the hospital. It is called *chelation* and it is a treatment that has been in use for some thirty years. Holistic doctors look upon it as a natural method of treatment for these illnesses.

Chelation means *binding*. It involves feeding substances like vitamin C or EDTA (an amino acid with the full name of ethylenediaminetetraacetic acid) directly into the veins through a standard hospital drip of the same type you will associate with intravenous feeding. The purpose of chelation is to improve circulation and remove toxic metals from the body. In the case of someone with severe circulatory problems, it can mean an alternative to surgery, which offers no guarantee of a long-term improvement in the majority of cases. And chelation comes without the risks and expense of vascular surgery.

Altogether some 70,000 people in the United States have coronary bypass surgery every year at an approximate cost of $12,000 each. The total annual cost to the health care system is approaching $1 billion, yet recurrence of symptoms is common even if initial results are satisfactory. What's more, the National Institute of Health reported in the New England Journal of Medicine in 1978, the recurrence of symptoms appears to be related to the progression of arteriosclerosis in the remaining ungrafted arteries. In other words, the arteries which are not treated continue to get clogged, so it is important to treat the cause and not the symptoms.

Why are these people not given chelation therapy instead? After all, it is the treatment of choice for arteriosclerosis in some European centers. It is difficult to give a clear answer. Holistic doctors can only assume that bypass surgery is a monster growing in the shape of millions of dollars worth of highly sophisticated equipment and research, along with specially trained surgeons and special units in hospitals all dependent on it financially. In order to justify the equipment, it seems that we must keep using it.

From the holistic casebook:

Helena, a 52-year-old department store clerk, went to see her doctor complaining of chest pain upon exertion. The pain seemed to be most severe when she climbed the stairs to her third-floor apartment, but because of her fear of doctors she waited until the pain was almost incapacitating before seeking medical counsel. A thorough evaluation by a cardiologist revealed angina pectoris (chest pain due to lack of oxygen to the heart). She was prescribed nitrates and Inderal (a beta blocker to slow down the heartbeat and improve its efficiency) and was told if her condition did not respond she would be a candidate for coronary-bypass surgery. After adequate clinical trial, her symptoms persisted and, faced with surgery, she sought an alternative approach. At the holistic clinic she was placed on a less than 10 percent fat diet, heavy in unrefined carbohydrates, given a walking schedule, and chelation therapy. After twenty-two treatments she was asymptomatic on climbing her stairs at home and did not require the use of any medication.

Holistic doctors can only hope that, as they have looked for alternatives, so will increasing numbers of other doctors, until the tide is gradually turned. Until then, at HMG clinics we shall, when appropriate, recommend that patients with circulatory problems not responding to diet and exercise have chelation therapy. Eighty percent of them show quite dramatic improvement after treatment.

EDTA is safer, research has shown, than taking aspirin. All that is required of a patient is that he or she spend three to four hours seated in a comfortable reclining chair to allow the solution to be slowly dripped into the veins. Just why it works is not entirely understood; study is continuing in an effort to clearly define its capabilities. Current medical opinion is that it cleanses and rejuvenates tired and hardened arteries, removing substances that build up inside them over the years. Furthermore, it helps clear up other illness such as heavy metal and lead poisoning—for which it is the treatment of choice—as well as some cases of rheumatoid arthritis.

From the holistic casebook:

Annie is an 86-year-old widow who came to the clinic complaining of high blood pressure, early signs of senility including difficulty remembering, headaches, and chronically cold hands and feet. She was on heavy doses of anti-hypertensive medication consisting of several different types of pills. She had been ill for many years with a progression in the severity of her symptoms. Thermograms and plethysmagraphs were performed which showed extensive peripheral vascular occlusive disease. A low-fat diet and walking schedule were recommended along with a series of chelation treatments, twenty in all. By the tenth of them her systolic blood pressure dropped 30 millimeters with a ten-point drop in her diastolic pressure—a significant improvement on the level achieved by her medication. Between the fifteenth and twentieth chelation this patient's thinking became greatly improved with a dramatic increase in her energy level. Her own words were that she could hardly remember the last time she had felt so good, and was able to significantly reduce the level of medication she had been taking prior to the treatment.

Reggie, a 37-year-old college professor with a history of diabetes, was on 40 units of Lente U 100 insulin daily. He had an ulcer on his right foot that would not heal as a result of his diabetes. After treatment by two

dermatologists without success he consulted the
HMG. Evaluation revealed him to be a poorly controlled diabetic with peripheral vascular occlusive
disease (poor circulation in his extremities). He was
placed on a 10 percent fat, 50 percent unrefined carbohydrate diet and was given a therapeutic dose of
zinc and vitamins A, C and D. Combined with this he
was administered intravenous chelation therapy and
by the eighteenth treatment his ulcer was healed.
After twenty-five treatments his need for insulin had
been reduced by half.

The HMG doctors also use an intravenous drip to treat
severe allergies, severe colds and other illnesses. In these
treatments the solution contains vitamin C and is referred to
as megavitamin therapy (that is, doses of vitamins high above
the Recommended Daily Allowances). In the past few years
megavitamin therapy has aroused controversy, mainly because of the claims of some physicians that it acts as a cure-
all. Holistic doctors do not support this claim but they do not
subscribe to the contention of traditional physicians that it is
a worthless therapy. The HMG stands in the middle, feeling
that in some areas of illness, due to the individual nature of
body chemistries, additional vitamins can bring about considerable relief and prevention.

HMG physicians, in conjunction with Nobel laureate Dr.
Linus Pauling, feel all humans have a natural vitamin C deficiency because of an enzyme abnormality which inhibits its
manufacture in the body. It is possible to give it in tablet
form, but the intestines can only absorb so much. In some in-
stances vitamin C is fed directly into the veins in doses as
high as 50,000 mg. Use of megavitamins fulfills the need for
greater amounts of vitamins and minerals in some people due
to biochemical individuality, and compensates for the loss of
nutrients from food processing and storage. Indeed, it has

been found in our clinics that many people do not get even the Recommended Daily Allowances of vitamins in their diet. What must be remembered is that the RDA's were calculated as the amount necessary to exist, not necessarily to be well and wholly alive.

Gourmet Dining—American Style

"Hey, OK," cries Dad. "It's gonna be a treat. C'mon, you kids. We're eating out today."

So goes the call in American homes when Saturday rolls around. Mom gets a day away from the stove after a week of cooking for Dad and the kids, and the whole family gets together for what's easily the most popular weekend pastime around.

"Where are we going?" cries one of the delighted youngsters.

"Yes, where, where?" pleads the other.

It doesn't take Dad long to decide. Every night of the week he has seen the TV ads telling him where "the burgers are best," so he bundles his family into the car and a few minutes later they arrive outside the restaurant.

The hostess welcomes them and shows them to a lushly padded family booth that immediately has the kids thinking this is really something special. Even the menus are an attraction. They're big, colorful and gimmicky, with hamburgers dressed up a dozen different ways as well as lots of other entrees, soups and desserts.

"Wow, what a choice!" exclaims Junior. "What am I going to have out of all this." He ponders, and Dad eventually has to remind him that the waitress is poised over the table, pen and pad ready for the order.

Dad decides on the half-pounder, while Mom decides a four-ounce burger will be just right for her appetite. The youngsters get the "kids' specials" and Dad says they will have them all with french fries, a side order of salad, coffee, with soda pop for Junior and his brother.

Before they can say "Jack Robinson", the drinks in those amazing unbreakable mugs arrive. Minutes later, the waitress appears with food that's steaming cheerfully on the very latest in throw-away plates.

Dad's mouth waters, the kids shout "yum, yum," and Mom gets first choice of the impressive array of condiments on the table. She applies mustard generously to the meat, then pickles, and, just before the salt and pepper, a shake of thin brown seasoning sauce that she remembers makes a great clam dip. Dad decides on a dollop of steak sauce that "even makes burgers taste good" while the youngsters go eagerly for tomato ketchup. The clatter of this family's knives and forks join the happy cacophony that is "eating for fun."

Ten minutes later it is all over. The high of the hamburger becomes a low and Mom thinks those desserts look tempting indeed. The kids readily agree and while they attack apple pie a la mode, Dad gets the bill, tips the waitress and gives the change from $20 to the kids so they can buy some candy and chewing gum for the detour to the park on the way home.

Now you might ask, "What was wrong with all of that?" It sounded like traditional family life and good clean fun. But we set up the fictional situation so that you could understand a few less obvious truths about the American way of eating.

Let's look at it again. In fact, the whole thing has more to do with getting as much of Dad's money as possible than with nourishing the body, the real object of eating. It makes no sense to spend money for food and not only get no nutritional value from it, but have to pay the doctor to help relieve your upset stomach and high blood pressure and the dentist to fill cavities. By taking responsibility for what you put into your mouth, you can often keep from making yourself ill.

Look at the nutritional value of the meal itself. It's a bun, ground meat, lettuce, a slice of tomato, french fried potatoes and a few other edibles. The meat is protein but even the leanest ground beef can contain up to 30 percent fat and therefore is inadvisable in a good eating plan. The tomato and lettuce are good but their quantity will only make a small contribution to the vitamin and mineral needs of the average American. The bun is made out of bleached white flour, and the potatoes have been robbed of natural taste and nutrients by peeling and frying.

Do you see now why you need all those condiments to give this "treat" some taste. Over the years you've gotten used to burgers spread with mustard, or french fries smothered in ketchup, and the mustard and ketchup are all your taste buds are experiencing. But those condiments have no nutrient value.

Now we turn to the desserts. Unless you eat fresh fruit or natural yogurt, more than likely your dessert will contain surprising amounts of sugar and fat. Yet how many times have you indulged in your favorite ice cream and looked upon it as something you have earned as a treat? Many people eat ice cream every day. Perhaps they would not if they knew it contained more than 50 percent fat and sugar merely disguised with artificial vanilla or chocolate or other flavoring. The pie is the same. There's sugar in the crust, which is made from bleached white flour and fat, and there is sugar in the fruit filling, too. Whether you're weight watching or not, the heavy calorie count is not worth the smattering of nutrients you are getting. Soda pop comes into the same category. If it's "diet soda" it probably contains the artificial sweetener saccharin, which now carries a government health warning. If it isn't diet soda, it contains sugar by the spoonful and should be avoided.

Put those with the candy and chewing gum that Junior and his brother bought on the way out and you're really piling up the sugar. And do you really want to keep your youngsters quiet with sugar and chemicals? It also does not make economic sense if you equate the money spent with the amount of nutrition they provide. Once you realize what's in these foods, you will soon seek out different snacks for your children such as nuts, fruit, seeds, raisins and other natural goodies.

So there we have the family Saturday "treat". In a word, it was not far from "junk."

When holistic doctors start a diet evaluation, patients are asked to make up a 24-hour eating record. Do it yourself now, but don't forget to list all beverages, condiments, chewing gum, breath mints, candies, mustard, ketchup, salad dressing, butter and snacks. When you get to the end of the list, you'll surprise yourself. Not only will it no doubt consist of a whole array of useless, unnutritious foods, it will also show that you have been consuming too much as well, perpetuating indisputable correlation between a junk diet, obesity (60 percent of all Americans are more than 10 percent overweight) and sickness.

Consider these facts revealed by the Select Committee on Nutrition and Human Needs in their report in 1976 on "Diet and Killer Diseases," which support the statements made earlier in our discussion and explanation of the common chronic illnesses,

- "Six of the ten leading causes of death in the United States have been connected with diet—heart disease, cancer, stroke, hypertension, diabetes, arteriosclerosis, and cirrhosis of the liver."
- "Nutritional imbalances in the diet contribute to at least 30 percent of cancer cases in men and 50 percent in women."
- "In recent years it has become apparent that the best hope of achieving any significant extension of life expectancy lies in the area of *disease prevention.*"

- "Nutrition should be at least a primary component of a complete health care strategy, and the *most* basic constituent of *any* health promotion strategy."

    Therefore, in instructing patients in the prevention and treatment of chronic illnesses holistic doctors look closely at both the foods patients eat and the amounts.
    The following guide will provide you with a quick basic holistic eating summary. It will give you a general idea of what a healthy diet should be like.

Eat mostly:

Fresh vegetables, raw whenever possible.
    Fresh fruits.
Fruit and vegetable juices (unsweetened).
Raw cheese, yogurt, kefir and other raw, unpasteurized dairy products.
Raw nuts, seeds, sprouted seeds and beans.
Herb teas, bottled, distilled or spring water.
Fish, poultry, other white meats.
Whole grain breads and cereals.

Eat sparingly:

Animal proteins—especially limit beef.
Eggs.
Natural sweeteners such as unfiltered and uncooked honey, molasses and maple syrup.
Small quantities of sea salt or powdered kelp.
Natural herbs and spices.
Small quantities of butter and unrefined olive oil for cooking.
Unrefined cold-pressed oils for salads.

Do not eat:

All refined and or processed foods, which includes refined sugars, flours, rices and *all* junk food.

Coffee, decaffeinated coffee, regular tea, chocolate, soft and diet drinks, alcohol, beer.

Foods containing artificial flavorings and colorings.

Black pepper, creamy salad dressings, ketchup, steak sauce.

Margarine (which is an artifical food full of stabilizers, texturizers, artificial flavorings and colorings).

"White" foods (flour, sugar, rice, except naturally white foods e.g. milk—most have been bleached and robbed of nutrients by processing.

Ice cream.

Cake mixes.

Jello.

Bakery goods (except whole grain breads).

Candies and gum.

Mints (including "breath fresheners").

Lozenges.

Mouth wash.

Jam or jelly, processed.

Luncheon meats (salami, hot dogs, bologna).

Artificial sweeteners.

All medicines containing aspirin such as Bufferin, Anacin, Excedrin, Alka-Seltzer. Use Datril or Tylenol for pain or fever.

Do not use:

Toothpaste and toothpowder. (A mixture of salt and soda or naturally flavored clay and sea salt brands available from health stores can be used as substitutes.) Do not use perfumes (the chemicals they consist of can trigger sensitivities).

Holistic Tips:

• Check *all* labels of prepared or packaged foods and drugs for artificial coloring and flavoring.
• Omit *all* foods and drinks with chemical additives.

- Eat in moderation. Do *not* overeat—it is very stressful to the body.
- Always eat slowly and chew food well.
- Rotate foods to create a balanced diet and to avoid building up sensitivities.
- Avoid canned foods, if possible.

You will see that absent from the holistic eating list are the majority of the 50,000 items stocked by the average supermarket. That is because eating is really a simple business. There just aren't thousands of natural basic foods, nor do there need to be. Processed foods have been introduced to meet the demands of shoppers always wanting something new. Doubtless the increase of fad foods will go on unless you, the consumer, voice your objections and demand good food value for your money. Supermarkets, like fast-food restaurants, have only one objective in mind—profit. You have to determine if they deserve it. Remember, it is your job, not theirs, to make sure your body gets the nutrition it needs.

As our guideline for good eating indicated, it is better to avoid processed foods altogether. If a food has to be processed to preserve it or make it tastier, then it shouldn't be eaten. Many vitamins and minerals are lost during processing. That is bad for you and your body's needs, but okay with the manufacturer. It means his product can sit on the shelf longer, like the burger in the fast food restaurant. Although it might be labelled as a "convenience food", the convenience is the manufacturer's, not yours. The same is true of canned and frozen foods. Besides the lost nutrients in canned meat, fruit and vegetables, people can absorb high levels of toxic metal in their bodies from the can linings.

Naturally the more nutrients a meal can give you, the better it is for your body. Because of our poor dietary habits, the nutrients that people seem to lack most are vitamins. They probably should have been called "*vital*-mins"; the average

eater would then have attached much more importance to
them than he does now. A vitamin deficiency can have serious results, so every holistic eater should educate himself
about where these mysterious "vitals" come from.

Vitamin	Result of Deficiency	Good Sources
Vitamin A	Increased suscep-tibility to infection. Abnormal function of gastro-intes-tinal, urinary and respiratory tracts. Skin dries, shrivels, thickens. Night blindness. In severe cases, certain eye disease and other local infec-tions.	Animal fats, butter, cheese, cream, egg yolk, whole milk. Fish liver oil. Liver. Green leafy vegetables, especially kale and parsley. Yellow vegetables, especially carrots.
Thiamin (Vitamin B_1)	Loss of appetite. Impaired digestion of starches and sugars. Colitis, constipa-tion or diarrhea. Emaciation. In severe cases, nervous disorders of various types or loss or coor-dinating power of muscles. Beri-beri.	Whole grain cereals, peas, beans, peanuts, oranges, heart, liver, kidney, vegetables, fruits, nuts. In high con-centration in brewer's yeast.

Riboflavin (Vitamin B$_2$)	Impaired growth. Weakness and tiredness. Anemia. Cataracts. Cheilosis (lip disease). Glossitis (inflammation of the tongue). Sensitivity to light (photophobia).	Eggs, green vegetables, liver, kidney, lean meat, milk, wheat germ, yeast.
Niacin	Gastrointestinal disturbances. Pellagra (skin eruption). Mental disturbances.	Yeast, lean meat, fish, legumes, whole grain cereals, peanuts.
Vitamin B$_{12}$	Severe anemia.	Liver, kidney, dairy products.
Vitamin C	Lowered resistance to infections and colds. Joint tenderness. Susceptibility to dental decay pyorrhea and bleeding gums. In severe cases, hemorrhage, anemia or scurvy.	Abundant in most fresh fruits and vegetables, especially citrus fruits and juices, tomatoes and oranges.
Vitamin D	Irritability. Weakness. Interference with utilization of	Butter, egg yolk, fish, liver oils, salmon, tuna, herring, sardines,

	calcium and phosphorus in bone and teeth formation. In severe cases, rickets in young children.	liver, oysters, yeast. Also formed in the skin by exposure to sunlight.
Vitamin E	Red blood cell resistance to rupture is decreased	Lettuce, green leafy vegetables, wheat germ oil, brown rice.
Vitamin B_6	Dermatitis around eyes and mouth. Anorexia (absence of appetite). Nausea and vomiting. Neuritis (a nervous disorder).	Blackstrap molasses, meat, cereal grains, wheat germ.
Folic Acid	Anemia.	Green leafy vegetables, yeast, glandular meats.

It will be evident that the enemy of the dieter, fat, has not been eliminated completely from the chart. Fat in moderation is beneficial to the body.

Why cannot fat be cut out completely? Your body must absorb nutrients from fat sources to maintain quality and tone of the skin and hair; and, of course, we all need a thin layer of fat around our bodies to protect and cushion the organs inside. It is better, however, to eat fatty foods in the morning, as they take longer to be broken down inside the body than nonfatty foods, and this process is best achieved during the day's activity.

Butter is one of the most common fats that we use daily in our diet. It is fine to use in moderation, but most avid butter eaters have to be careful of cholesterol levels building up in the blood. Both cheese and milk contain similar types of fat and if these are overlooked, even though little butter is consumed, the total cholesterol level can rise. Vegetable fats should be restricted, too. Current research seems to indicate that a fat is a fat and its source doesn't make any difference.

Holistic patients are advised not to drink coffee because it contains the drug caffeine. Caffeine is a stimulant which gives the body a "lift." This is caused by energy-giving glucose being shot into the blood stream, and thus a "high" is achieved, aided by an additional secretion of adrenalin, and the coffee drinker feels elated. In reality, the body in its natural state prefers an even keel and fights the lift the coffee produces, making you want another cup. If you charted your coffee consumption throughout the day, you would get a "hills and valleys" effect characteristic of addiction. It is quite ironic to hear people scoffing at the alcoholic or the chain-smoker when in fact they could be, as heavy coffee drinkers, equally hooked on caffeine. Coffee is nothing less than legalized "speed." Tea drinkers need not be complacent either. Caffeine is present in tea and in colas. It can cause pains like heartburn, which is an irritation in the gastrointestinal tract, and more seriously, raising of the blood pressure.

"But coffee, tea and colas are cornerstones of the American way of life," many patients complain. Their lives, like that of our character in the opening chapter, revolve around caffeine beverages; we hear many people exclaim that they'll give up everything else but "never my coffee." All the doctor can say is that it is making you ill gradually; rather than relieving stress with the "highs," it is an added stress for the body that will take its toll in the long run. Why not try a week or two on some other drink such as an herb tea and make it a challenge to break the coffee habit? There are many natural flavors and you will find their aroma and taste a whole new experience for you. Or try drinking broths or protein mixtures that any health food store sells. They are made from natural roots, berries or beans and make a welcome change.

Fruit juices have become victims of big business. Over the years they have gone from fresh-squeezed fruits and berries to artificially flavored, artificially colored bottles of sugared water. These are in no way nutritious and should be avoided. The only acceptable juices are those squeezed fresh, so buy the oranges and squeeze them yourself. Many juicers today will take the whole fruit, extracting every drop of nutrition from an orange, a carrot, an apple, or anything else that takes your fancy. Because nothing goes to waste, it can be extremely economical too.

The question of seasonings and other supplementary foods like candy and alcohol also arises when considering optimal health. Too much salt can raise blood pressure and cause fluid retention. Too much pepper can irritate the stomach lining and bring on gastric distress. Many people have become so accustomed to seasoning food in this way that they have lost the real taste of food. Garlic, which is a natural and nutritious food would be far better to use when seasoning is required. Generally, anything that is craved and consumed on a daily basis will be causing some problem somewhere inside the body. (As we already know, excessive sugar consumption brings on hypoglycemia and adult onset diabetes.) With chocolate it could be acne or migraine; if it is alcohol, the trouble could be more serious. Bear in mind that just as you can be an alcoholic, you can be a sugarholic too.

If you are a chocolate lover, try carob, which is not only similar in taste and appearance, but is highly nutritious too. Or if you like vanilla, try the natural, real thing instead of the chemical vanillin which is used in many ice creams, sauces and candies. Almost all flavorings originated with natural substances in Grandma's day and it is a pleasant (and healthy) exercise to go back to the originals.

Bread, rice, and red meat are essentially nutritious foods, but processing reduces their nutritional benefits immensely. Today, bread and rice have to be "enriched" (vitamins have to be added by the manufacturer) because the processing they go through to make them more "convenient" for you strips them of their nutritious coating. These "enriched" foods still fall short of what the original whole grains and brown rice (as whole rice is known) can provide. They also lack fiber, which has virtually disappeared from the western diet due to refining. Fiber is cellulose unable to be digested by the body. As already mentioned in the discussion of chronic illnesses, diverticular disease can be caused by chronic constipation. And with this chronic constipation can occur waste putrifying in the colon, with increased likelihood of bowel cancer according to medical studies. This putrification is less toxic if there is adequate fiber in the diet, because the whole process of moving food through your body is speeded up. For those people, perhaps laxative users who feel they are getting insufficient fiber in their diet, a daily serving of unprocessed miller's bran may provide relief from constipation. Mix it with cereals, sprinkle it on food or take it in a glass of water—you will probably never need to spend money on laxatives again. The missing fiber in the American diet is one reason why you should switch to whole grains and brown rice. Another reason is the additional vitamins and minerals they provide naturally, without the need for enrichment.

Beef, pork and lamb are the meats that America has grown up on. But have we had too much of a good thing? Holistic doctors believe we have. In America, eating meat was once only something the wealthy could do. Even now in Europe, because of its price, a little meat must go a long way, and meals are made up with bread and vegetables. However, in the United States, meat has become a must on everyone's plate.

There appears to be a correlation between meat consumption and illness. Surveys of Seventh-Day Adventists, about half of whom are vegetarians, show that they suffer one-half the heart-attack deaths that other Americans do, have far lower death rates from breast and colon cancer and live longer.

The low quality of meat today is a problem; it has become too fatty, even though it is an excellent source of protein. The reason for this is the way the animals are fed and injected with chemicals and hormones to fatten them up in the last few weeks before slaughtering, thereby giving the farmer, the meat dealer and the middle-men higher profits. You may not be able to see the fat in your meat, but it is there in every strand.

A far better source of protein is white or game meat and fish which contain little fat. Into this category come veal, chicken, turkey, rabbit, pigeon, hare, venison and elk.

However, many people are unaware of how to cook them. It's easier than you think. Probably the best way is to experiment with wine, garlic and herbs—the secrets of gourmet cooking. Place the fish or meat in a casserole and add red or white wine, chopped clove of garlic for each serving and a sprinkle of herbs like oregano or basil. Mix with that the standard garnishes like scallions, onions, mushrooms, tomatoes, a few carrots and bake in a hot oven. And of course, always make sure the meat and fish are fresh, not frozen or canned.

If wine cookery does not appeal, or you feel experimenting will be too adventurous, the following measured recipes will be of help.

CHICKEN CASSEROLE

7 oz. chicken breast, boned and skinned
½ cup of celery, chopped
½ cup of tomato, chopped
2 tbs. of parsley, chopped
Bay leaf, pinch of thyme
1 cup of broth or stock, low fat
1 cup of fresh mushrooms, chopped

Brown chicken in pan glazed with French diet dressing. Transfer to casserole and add celery, tomato, parsley, bay

leaf, thyme, broth. Cover and bake at 350 degrees for 45
minutes. Add mushrooms and cook for 15 minutes. Remove
bay leaf. Makes two servings.

STEAMED CHICKEN OR FISH

Place meat in foil, completely sealed and bake in oven. To
chicken add:
    either sliced celery
           soy sauce
           sage
      or orange juice
           2 drops angostura bitters
           ginger

Bake at 400 degrees for 30 to 40 minutes.

To fish add:
    either bay leaf
           chopped parsley
           lemon juice
      or 1 tbs. French diet dressing
           paprika
      or diet tomato juice
           herbs

Bake at 350 degrees for 25 minutes.

TWO-IN-ONE

Can be prepared with either chicken breast or veal.
    3½ oz. of flattened chicken breast or veal cut into strips.
    1 cup of tomato, chopped
    Clove of garlic
    Pinch of oregano and black pepper
    1 slice of bell pepper

Broil meat until tender. Mash tomatoes and add to pan. Add the balance of seasonings. Place meat in pan and simmer for 10 minutes.

VEAL STEAK SWISS

7 oz. veal steak, all fat removed
2 tomatoes, blanched, peeled, cut up
Bay leaf, dash of thyme
1 clove of garlic
½ cup of stock

Brown meat well in pan glazed with a little French diet dressing. Add rest of ingredients. Simmer, covered, for one hour at 350 degrees. Serves two.

VEAL KEBAB

½ oz. cubed veal (or chicken or fish)
½ cup whole mushrooms
½ cup cherry tomatoes
Lemon juice

Marinate meat in Italian diet dressing thinned with a little lemon juice for several hours or overnight. Arrange on skewers alternating mushrooms and tomatoes. Broil until brown, turning several times.

BROILED LEAN FISH

3½ oz. fish fillet
Clove garlic
Juice of one lemon

Sprinkle fillets with seasonings. Brush on lemon juice. Broil until fish flakes easily with fork.

BREADSTICK FISH

3½ oz. fish fillet
Juice of one lemon
1 breadstick (or breadcrumbs), whole grain

Crush breadstick into crumbs and season with rosemary to taste. Dry fish fillet with a paper towel and brush with lemon juice. Roll in seasoned breadcrumbs. Broil until tender.

BAKED CRAB AND TOMATO

3½ oz. of crab meat
1 cup of chopped tomatoes
2 tbs. chopped parsley
1 slice of onion
Juice of one lemon

Bake in small baking dish at 325 degrees until tender.

CURRIED SHRIMP OR CRAB

2 tbs. French diet dressing
½ tsp. curry powder (or to taste)
Raisins (handful)
3½ oz. shrimp or crab

HOT: Heat dressing and seasonings in sauce pan (add a small amount of water if desired). Toss with hot cooked shrimp or crab and raisins and serve on a bed of cooked bean sprouts.

COLD: Mix dressing and seasonings together and toss with cold cooked shrimp or crab and raisins. Chill and serve on bed of lettuce.

BAKED HALIBUT STEAK

3½ oz. halibut steak
½ tsp. dry mustard
Dash of tarragon
Juice of one lemon

Sprinkle halibut steak with seasonings and lemon juice. Bake at 350 degrees in foil until tender.

SHELLFISH MANDARIN

1 clove of garlic, chopped
2 cups of bean sprouts or celery or asparagus pieces
1 tbs. green onion, chopped
⅓ cup of hot water and juice of ½ lemon
1 tbs. soy sauce
7 oz. lobster or shrimp
Pinch of basil or chervil

Saute garlic, green onion and lobster or shrimp in pan glazed with diet dressing over low heat for 15 minutes. Add bean sprouts, water, soy sauce and simmer for about 5 minutes. (For asparagus, add with fish and onion) Serves two.

FISH SPECIAL

Used for haddock, flounder, sole, shrimp, crab or lobster.
3½ oz. of fish
1 cup of tomatoes, chopped
1 slice of onion, chopped
1 slice of bell pepper
1 bay leaf
2 tbs. chopped parsley

½ cup of water
1 clove garlic, chopped

Simmer tomatoes with all ingredients except fish for 10 minutes. Add fish and cook until tender.

Fruits and vegetables form an integral part of eating the holistic way. Certainly, as eating habits stand at the moment, we do not get enough of either. We know fruits and vegetables are beneficial and answer many of the demands of a holistic diet. Properly grown and fresh, they are packed with vitamins and minerals and should, if possible, be eaten several times per day. It is an all too common sight to see the vegetables served with an expensive restaurant meal pushed to the side of the plate by the diner who believes the meat is more important to his body. When you're eating out, demand fresh vegetables. Frozen and canned foods lose many of their nutrients and suffer dismally in taste. Yet they are an easy compromise for restaurants—they'll keep for a long time and are always on hand, regardless of supply and demand. That is not good enough. You are the money end of the deal, so demand, and make sure you get, only the best. Inquire before you order and if the vegetables are not fresh, exercise your prerogative and leave. Find another restaurant and tell a friend. If enough pressure is applied, the situation will soon change.

If you decide that home is the place to discover the joys of vegetables, try eating them separate from the main course, as those experts in cuisine, the French, do. But do not overcook them; few vegetables need longer than ten minutes in boiling spring water with a clove of chopped garlic to taste. Then serve them with a tiny pat of butter.

Fruit and nuts are a marvelous way to break the snack habit. If you feel you must have a mint, a candy, or gum during the day, try having a banana, pear, grapes or plain unsalted nuts instead. Again, they contain many of the nutrients you need. Soon you will wonder how you could possibly have preferred foods that depend upon artificial colors, flavors and much sugar. Read the labels and generally anything ending in *-ose* is a sugar of one form or another, such as dextrose or sucrose. Fruit contains its own natural sugar, but in the form of fructose, which is readily absorbed as energy by the body. However, too much of a good thing can be bad, and the best way to make sure you are not overdoing it is to eat no more than three or four pieces of fruit daily. All things in moderation is the key to a good, healthy diet.

Learning how to eat in a new way is not just a matter of finding out which foods are good and which foods are bad. It is necessary to combine your foods properly so that optimum digestion inside the stomach can take place. Certain combinations of food do not digest well together and can contribute to problems with indigestion, bloating, belching, heartburn, flatulence, or abdominal discomfort. The chart on the following page gives you an idea of good food combinations.

Drinking excessive amounts of liquids with meals is another habit worth looking at. It's customary to have a beverage with lunch or dinner. If the fare is hamburger and French fries or other greasy food, it is often needed to "wash it down." But liquids during a meal dilute the gastric juices in the stomach, so it is more advisable to drink 10-15 minutes before the meal. The best way to break the habit is to drink water at regular intervals during the day. This practice, combined with better food, will make it unnecessary to drink beer, soda or milk during meals.

For many people, the changes outlined will be radical, but for others who may have been drifting in the right direction as a result of greater awareness of the problems of today's diet, they will be welcome guidelines. If at all possible, have your diet individualized by a physician or qualified nutritionist. Some people need more of allowable foods, while others can get by on less depending on the functioning and chemistry of their body. As a rule of thumb proportion your food so that your total diet consists of 50 percent unrefined carbohydrates, 30 percent protein, and 20 percent fat.

FOOD-COMBINING FOR BETTER DIGESTION

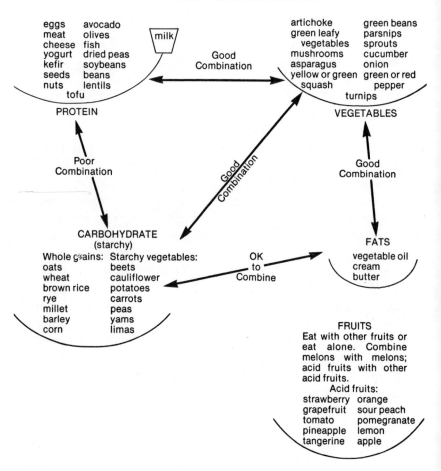

eggs	avocado
meat	olives
cheese	fish
yogurt	dried peas
kefir	soybeans
seeds	beans
nuts	lentils
	tofu

PROTEIN

milk

Good Combination

artichoke	green beans
green leafy	parsnips
vegetables	sprouts
mushrooms	cucumber
asparagus	onion
yellow or green	green or red
squash	pepper
	turnips

VEGETABLES

Poor Combination

Good Combination

Good Combination

Good Combination

CARBOHYDRATE
(starchy)

Whole grains:	Starchy vegetables:
oats	beets
wheat	cauliflower
brown rice	potatoes
rye	carrots
millet	peas
barley	yams
corn	limas

OK to Combine

FATS
vegetable oil
cream
butter

FRUITS
Eat with other fruits or eat alone. Combine melons with melons; acid fruits with other acid fruits.
Acid fruits:

strawberry	orange
grapefruit	sour peach
tomato	pomegranate
pineapple	lemon
tangerine	apple

Holistic Tips:
- Three or four different foods per meal are plenty.
- Eat only one concentrated protein food per meal if possible.
- Drink liquids 10–15 minutes before meals or several hours afterwards or small amount with meals.
- Try to have at least three hours between meals.
- Sweets like honey do not digest well with proteins or carbohydrates.

From the holistic casebook:

Elizabeth is an 18-year-old, working at the check-out of a supermarket. She has had a history of skin rashes after eating sugar, honey, dairy products and drinking coffee. She also complained of an inability to sleep and frequent muscle pains. (Her ailments might appear on the severe side for one so young, but, in fact, this condition is increasingly common in teen-agers. Holistic doctors greatly attribute it to an inadequate diet and excessive junk food and soda pop.) The patient was put through extensive food allergy testing and was found to be sensitive to a vast variety of foods. Rather than take her off all these foods, a program was established to gradually eliminate them. She was also instructed on how to properly combine her foods and rotate them to help avoid flareups in her skin condition. Elizabeth immediately felt a resurgence of energy after some of the offending foods had been removed from her diet. Her skin condition, however, did not respond until several weeks later by which time it began to lose its dry texture and assumed a healthy glow. She was further advised to restrain use of facial cosmetics which she had been in the habit of using to cover her rash. The diet change was also coupled with vitamin and mineral supplements which alleviated her muscle pains and enabled her to double her sleep time and to date none of her problems have recurred.

A Weighty Problem?

Without doubt, obesity is a national epidemic so rampant that it has become a social problem of our times. Thirty-three percent of the patients going through the HMG are up to 15 percent above their ideal weight. Though each individual differs, reducing can be a relatively simple matter. A sensible program of eating and exercise will soon take off extra pounds.

Obesity, however, is a different problem. Using 15 percent above ideal weight as the dividing line, many people are found to be obese, and some are more than twice their optimum weight. Scientists have estimated that the excess energy consumed by this nation's fat people would be enough to provide domestic power to several large cities. The calculation was made by the University of Illinois' Energy Research Group and reported in the American Journal of Public Health. They used data from the 1975 National Health Survey that found there was a staggering 1.5 billion pounds of excess fat on American women and an equally amazing 850 million pounds excess on the men. Converted to calories, which are units of energy, it would mean a saving of 5.7 trillion calories *daily* if each of the 50 million fat men and the 60 million fat women reduced their daily intake by just 600 calories. The scientists then converted those saved calories to thermal units and found that the saving would power the residential demands of San Francisco, Boston, Chicago and Washington.

In the past few years there has been an awakening of public opinion against obesity, but there is still a long way to go. Hopefully, the thinking behind holistic health will make a significant contribution.

Losing weight is not just a matter of starving the body of food so that it burns up its own fat. Once a diet course has been completed, the dieter often will relax and regain the weight. Most weight loss clinics throughout the country are seeing the same patients time and time again. The key to losing weight is in the mind. That is where the desire for food starts. Once that is controlled, weight gain will not take place.

In order to achieve a state of mind that controls weight, it is necessary to find out why you overeat. There are many different reasons why people are fat and if you check off, on the following questionnaire, those that apply to you, you will have a better idea of why you are overweight.

1. I eat quickly.
2. I eat in many rooms in the house.
3. I eat meals and snacks at irregular hours.
4. I don't talk to others during meals.
5. I do other things while I eat (watch TV, read).
6. I keep high-calorie foods around the house.
7. I don't pay much attention to what or how much I am eating.
8. I don't plan meals in advance for calorie content.
9. I take large portions when being served.
10. I often eat alone.
11. I overeat when I am depressed or worried.

12. Food calms me when I am nervous.
13. I get irritable or argumentative when I am hungry or on a diet.
14. I am not happy unless I feel full after a meal.
15. I get excited when I plan to eat a high-calorie meal or my favorite snack.
16. Eating takes my mind off my problems.
17. I eat more when I am angry at myself or someone else.
18. I eat more when I am tired.
19 I feel better after I eat.
20. I overeat when I am frustrated.
21. I always feel hungry.
22. My muscles get tense when I'm hungry.
23. I lose control when I smell food cooking.
24. I look at food a lot (in pictures, while shopping).
25. My stomach aches when I'm hungry.
26. I talk about or listen to conversations about food a great deal.
27. I get headaches, cramps, dizzy when I'm hungry.
28. My mouth waters when I see food I like.
29. I have no energy when I'm hungry.
30. I never feel full after a meal.
31. I get restless when I'm hungry.
32. I think more about food when I'm hungry or dieting.
33. I fantasize that I can eat all I want and never gain a pound.
34. When people talk about food, I can picture it in my imagination.
35. I think about food throughout the day.
36. I can't imagine what I would look like as a thin person.
37. Many of my fantasies are about food or eating.
38. When I fantasize, I think of myself as being thin and getting everything I want.
39. When I am hungry I dream about food and eating.
40. Sometimes I have thoughts about food that I cannot stop.
41. I have no will power.

42. Nothing is as satisfying as food.
43. I could never be or stay thin.
44. I can't give up my favorite foods.
45. Life would be perfect if I were thin.
46. I am overweight because of physical problems.
47. I can't be happy unless I eat all I want.
48. I don't deserve to be happy.
49. I am never going to be able to change.
50. It takes too much effort to be thin.
51. Thin people can eat whatever they want and not gain weight.
52. Some people prefer me overweight.
53. I can get even with people by being obese.
54. Most of my friends overeat or are obese.
55. Most of my social activities involve eating.
56. I am alone a great deal.
57. I enjoy eating more than talking to people.
58. I never get what I want from people.
59. My family will not help me lose weight.
60. If I lose weight, nobody will care.
61. Other people encourage me to eat.
62. I can dominate people by being big.
63. I am not an active person.
64. I do not care about wearing stylish clothes.
65. I drink or take drugs excessively.
66. I don't care what I look like when I go out.
67. I don't enjoy participation in sports.
68. I avoid appearing in a bathing suit.
69. I rarely buy clothes and don't enjoy shopping for clothes.
70. Other people think I am older than I really am.
71. I have more medical problems than most people.
72. I rarely try to make myself look attractive.

If you now go back over your answers you will be in a position to focus on where your particular reason for overeating lies. You will no doubt see that there are links in your behavior that give you characteristics normal-weight people do not have. That is precisely why they are thin. They will take out their frustrations in other ways—not by having a go at the bread loaf and jam jar. They will find other pleasures like walking which can be much more satisfying than eating. You have the reasons laid out in front of you. Now make the decision and resolve to change your thinking about food and eating. Use it as an exercise of mind over body. If you can get the right frame of mind now, you are already on the way to losing weight forever.

There are of course, physical reasons why some people put on weight. It can be malfunction in the glands or the digestive system and for these people—the minority of overweight people—a different course of treatment has to be followed. If you feel you are in this category, make sure you have had a diagnosis by a doctor to that effect. Some fat people have conditioned their minds to think that glandular malfunction is the reason they are overweight. They go through life eliciting sympathy from friends and relatives, when their real problem is simply overeating. Excuses among fat people abound, and for these people losing weight will be a lifelong business. It is reality that is called for, not fantasy, and if you can see that, it is not terribly difficult to start shedding pounds.

It is again a change in lifestyle that is demanded—a modification in your behavior. It is up to you how subtle or radical that change will be. Try not to worry about it, or make a bigger deal of it than it should be. Millions of other people do it naturally without prompting, so you can slip quietly in there with them. Gradually you will see your behavior change if you stick to these 20 golden rules.

1. In the supermarket, select only simple foods. Ignore the eye-level shelves.
2. Park away from the door and walk.
3. Shop from a list (make the list only *after* you have eaten).
4. Buy only nonfattening foods.
5. Buy poultry and fish and only the leanest cuts of meat.

6. Always have a variety of "safe" snack foods handy.
7. Buy with consideration for yourself and the health of your family.
8. Eat in only one room in the house.
9. Dine with someone when possible.
10. Engage in personal communication as the *only* other activity when you are eating.
11. Talk when there is no food in your mouth.
12. Slow down the rate of your eating.
13. Lay utensils down when you are chewing and swallowing.
14. Make portions appear larger by serving them on a smaller plate.
15. Add color to your meal (with green peas, orange, carrots) and make eating a pure experience.
16. Make second helpings hard to get.
17. Allow each member of the family to serve themselves and to remove their dishes from the table.
18. Do not skip meals. Plan and eat three meals daily.
19. When eating out, have an idea of what you want before you see the menu. Look at the menu and close it.
20. When dining at the home of friends, allow them to know that you practice preventive medicine and nutrition, and that you may eat small portions or refrain from eating certain foods with no disrespect to them.

Holistic Tips:

- Walk-stop saving steps.
- Take up a hobby.
- Introduce physical activity into your life at every opportunity.

The next step in weight reduction at holistic clinics involves the actual reduction in eating, which combines with what the patient now knows about his psychological condition. With the lessons learned, there is not too much difficulty embarking upon a food intake of about 1000 calories a day. It has to be as low as this because a fat body has to reduce itself from within and if it is constantly being resupplied at a normal rate, reduction will not occur.

It is possible to make a low-calorie diet filling by packing it with foods high in fiber. Vegetables are best for this; you will see from the following example of a holistic diet that there are plenty of good, low-calorie vegetables available.

Breakfast: Approximately 160 calories.

>   Choice of: ½ grapefruit *or* 1 small orange *or* 1 serving of melon *or* 4 oz. orange juice *or* 4 oz. grapefruit juice.
>   Plus choice of: 2–3 oz. nonsweetened whole grain or bran cereal *or* ½ cup cooked cereal.
>   Plus ½ cup skim milk
>   Plus 1 cup of herb tea

Lunch: Approximately 270 calories.

>   Choice of: 6 oz. tomato *or* vegetable juice.
>   Plus choice of: 4 oz. cottage cheese *or* 3 oz. chicken, boiled or broiled *or* 3 oz. broiled fish *or* 3 oz. salmon or tuna.
>   Plus choice of vegetables
>   1 slice of whole grain bread
>   1 cup of herb tea

Dinner: Approximately 500 calories.

>   Choice of: ½ grapefruit *or* ½ cantaloupe *or* 6 oz. tomato/vegetable juice.
>   Plus 6 oz. of chicken, boiled or broiled *or* 4 oz. broiled fish.
>   Plus choice of vegetables
>   herb tea

Daily Snacks

Choice of one—8 oz. skim milk, 8 oz. buttermilk, 6 oz.
plain low-fat yogurt, 3 oz. cottage cheese (approx.
90 calories).
Choice of two—1 apple, 1 cup strawberries, ½ can-
taloupe, ½ grapefruit, 1 cup cherries, 5 oz.
grapes, 1 orange, 2 peaches (approx. 70 calories).

Low-Calorie Vegetables (None over fifty calories)

cabbage	lettuce
carrots	onion
celery	radishes
cucumber	tomato
green or red pepper	sauerkraut

1 serving = 1 cup
approx. 20 calories each

artichokes	mushrooms
asparagus	okra
beets	spinach
broccoli	string beans
brussels sprouts	summer squash
cauliflower	turnips

1 serving = ½ cup
approx. 30 calories each

corn (1 ear, 5″ long)
green peas (½ cup)
parsnips (½ cup)
potato (1 medium, either baked or boiled)

approx. 50 calories each

Holistic tip:

Use low-calorie salad dressing or lemon juice as gar-
nish.

It should be pointed out at this stage that if you are severely overweight, it is not advisable to diet without first consulting a doctor. One of the main reasons is that apart from the behavior modification and the diet, permanent weight loss can only be achieved with exercise as well. As obese people tend not to have well-exercised bodies, any physical exertion or stress from dieting could adversely affect the heart.

Patients at the HMG clinics diet under close supervision of both the doctor and the paramedical staff; they also often attend discussion groups to talk over their progress. They are encouraged to keep workbooks of exactly what they are eating and doing during their time at home and this helps toward the sort of mental discipline necessary in permanent weight loss. It has to be remembered that few patients are *only* overweight. In most cases they have other chronic illnesses to be dealt with—this is why there is no one specific diet that can be used. A patient with high cholesterol levels may need a much different diet from someone with ulcers.

The foods that all dieters eat do have a similarity. They are low in fat. Since they also come into the eating plan of all holistic patients, only in larger quantities, it is worth having a checklist handy as you can see just how many calories they each comprise.

	Meat/Fish	*Calories*
chicken	1 breast, 8 oz., boned	210
veal	4 oz.	198
chicken livers	3½ oz.	141
clams	4 oz.	80
crab	3 oz.	86
lobster	3 oz.	80
mussels	6 medium	75
shrimp	3 oz.	100
albacore	3 oz., drained	170
bluefish	4 oz., baked or broiled	180
butterfish	3 oz.	176

catfish	3 oz.	168
flounder	4 oz.	78
halibut	4 oz.	228
perch	4 oz.	80
trout	3 oz.	60

	Vegetables	*Calories*
artichokes	4 hearts	20
asparagus	1 cup spears	36
bamboo shoots	3½ oz.	27
string beans	½ cup	35
bean sprouts	½ cup	15
broccoli	1 cup	44
brussels sprouts	1 cup	44
cabbage	1 cup	24
celery	1 cup	27
cauliflower	1 cup	30
chard	1 cup	30
collards	1 cup	76
kale	8 oz.	45
lettuce	1 lb. head	68
mushrooms, fresh	1 cup	20
spinach	1 cup	22
zucchini	4 oz.	23

	Fruit	*Calories*
apple	1	76
apricots	3	54
cantaloupe	½	37
grapefruit	½	75
orange	1	70
papaya	8 oz.	71
peach	1	46
pear	1	95
pineapple	8 oz.	74
strawberries	8 oz.	54

Bread		Calories
breadstick	1	20
melba toast	1 piece	20
cracked wheat	½ slice	40
whole wheat	½ slice	27

Holistic Tips:

- Control your food intake both in quantity (by measure) and in frequency (by time).
- If you are on a diet, be sure other family members who are directly involved with your eating (shopping, food preparation) understand and are willing to cooperate.
- Also elicit the help of others to cooperate with you concerning activities that are incompatible with your eating plans.
- Avoid having others run errands for you—be the first to jump when any errand is needed.
- Move items out of the kitchen which are incompatible with eating, such as the telephone, radio or television.
- Avoid using the kitchen table for reasons other than eating meals (arts and crafts, reading the paper).
- When the weather is nice, take indoor activities outside away from the kitchen (reading material, hobbies, sewing, television or radio).
- Until you are firmly in control of your eating habits, avoid social gatherings where you are uncomfortable without eating or drinking.
- The next time you bend over for something, leave it there and bend over again to pick it up.

There are now just two more factors to be dealt with in attaining a full holistic life. They are management of stress (referred to earlier as being a major factor in the causes of many chronic illnesses) and exercise. Most of us have too much of the former to do too little of the latter. This section is designed to give you guidelines for correcting those imbalances within the framework of your new lifestyle. What has been achieved so far are brand new eating habits and an awareness of the foods and products that are both good and bad for your body. Now you need to make adaptions in your life which will ensure that those advantages gained will be sustained.

Time Running Out?

Walk outside early in the morning virtually anywhere in the United States and you would be forgiven for thinking the whole world had gone jogging crazy. Joggers come young, old, and everywhere in between. It seems as though the streets and parks have become running tracks for physical fitness fanatics. But in fact that is a warped impression, because only a small percentage of the population gets sufficient exercise to give them a protection against illness. In the HMG clinics, more than 95 percent of new patients—a staggeringly high figure—have no regular exercise program. For many, the most strenuous thing they do all day is walk to the car or pick up a shopping bag. Think for a moment how much exercise you get. You take elevators instead of stairs, use the car instead of walking, have every labor-saving de-

---

Liberal use of material contained in the excellent booklet entitled *Beyond Diet . . . Exercise Your Way to Fitness and Heart Health* by Lenore R. Zohman, M.D. (published as a public service by the Mazola Corn Oil division of Best Foods, Copyright © 1974 by CPC International, Inc., Englewood Cliffs, NJ) has been made throughout this chapter.

vice possible inside and outside the house, and probably do not own any sort of exercising apparel that you could use even if you wanted to do something strenuous. But the problem appears to be more than lack of incentive on the part of patients. The average general practitioner could be just as much to blame. A Harris poll of doctors in late 1978 came up with the surprising revelation that most physicians rarely mention health and exercise in the same breath when seeing their patients. In fact, the correlation is so nonexistent that it led Dr. Stephen Hedberg, a clinical professor of surgery at Harvard University, to write in all seriousness in a *Medical World News* article: "It's not bad advice (on exercise) people are getting from doctors—it's no advice."

"My golf," you say, or "my tennis". Fine, but they do not provide the sort of exercise that will give any protection to your heart. And that is the number-one priority because, as we know, heart disease accounts for *more than 50 percent* of all deaths. Several studies at this time seem to indicate that exercise will provide some protection against heart disease; it also serves as a natural form of relaxation and stress reducer.

The cardinal rule you must understand and accept is: *Exercise is as important a part of your life as eating and sleeping.* Despite the temptations and pressures from the automobile, transportation and gadget industries, you must exercise regularly and keep it up throughout your life. A basic decision to do so is needed now in order to change your life successfully. If you can make that decision you are already halfway there, but be sure it is a firm resolve. If you are not so sure, consider this: Paying your physical dues need take no longer than one hour a day. And when you can do it with ease, it is unlikely you will be overweight again—not to mention as free from illness as is possible.

The rewards are substantial for effort on your part. Try to make the change now. It doesn't matter whether you are 20 or 50 or 70. Exercise comes in prescription form, and by consulting a holistic doctor you will be getting the prescription that is tailor-made for you. This is important because, for certain people, exercise can be dangerous. In most cases it is advisable to consult a physician before beginning an exercise program, but it is doubly important if you come into the "dangerous" category. To find out whether or not you do, take a moment to answer the following 25 questions. If you mark a "yes" against any one of them, do not begin to exercise without having a complete medical checkup.

1. Has a doctor ever said you had heart trouble?
2. Have you ever had rheumatic fever, growing pains, twitching of the limbs called St. Vitus' dance, or rheumatic heart disease?
3. Did you ever have, or do you now have, a heart murmur?
4. Have you ever had a real or suspected coronary occlusion, myocardial infarction, coronary attack, coronary insufficiency, heart attack or coronary thrombosis?
5. Do you have angina pectoris?
6. Have you ever had an abnormal electrocardiogram?
7. Have you ever had an electrocardiogram taken while you were exercising (such as climbing up and down steps) which was not normal?
8. Have you ever had pain or pressure of a squeezing feeling in the chest which came on during exercise or walking or any other physical or sexual activity?
9. If you climb a few flights of stairs fairly rapidly, do you have tightness or pressing pain in your chest?
10. Do you get pressure or pain or tightness in the chest if you walk in the cold wind or get a cold blast of air?
11. Have you had bouts of rapid heart action, irregular heart action or palpitations?
12. Have you ever taken digitalis, quinidine or any drug for your heart?
13. Have you ever been given nitroglycerin, sometimes labeled TNG or NTG, or any pills for chest

pain which you use by placing them under the tongue?

14. Do you have diabetes, high blood sugar or sugar in the urine now or at any time in the past?
15. Have you ever or do you now have high blood pressure or hypertension?
16. Have you been on a diet or taken medications to lower your blood cholesterol?
17. Are you more than 20 pounds heavier than you should be?
18. In your family has there been more than one heart attack, or coronary, or one person with heart trouble before age 60 (blood relative)?
19. Do you now smoke more than a pack and a half of cigarettes per day?
20. Do you have any chronic illnesses?
21. Do you have asthma, emphysema or other lung condition?
22. Do you get very short of breath from activities which don't make other people similarly short of breath?
23. Have you ever gotten, or do you now get, cramps in your legs if you walk several blocks?
24. Do you have arthritis, rheumatism, gout or gouty arthritis or a predisposition to gout? Has the uric acid in your blood been found to be high?
25. Do you have any condition limiting the motion of your muscles, joints, or any part of the body, which could be aggravated by exercise?

You will realize that the questions center mostly around the heart. The latter six were included because people with these ailments do better to seek out an exercise prescription, if only because they would find any form of activity strenuous. There is no better way to kill off desire than to get that "never again" feeling after your very first workout. People with chronic illnesses and people over 35 need to start exercising gradually and work up to a sustaining level, rather than risking the tragic consequences of an enthusiastic, breathless first try.

The point of that physical checkup is to measure the heart's and lungs' power and to determine your *aerobic* capacity. For most people that will be a new word. It is used frequently in the medical profession, particularly among doctors specializing in exercise, but it has not yet become common in everyday language. It comes from the word *aerobe*, which is a micro-organism requiring oxygen, or air, in order to live. The cells of your body come into that category; they must be constantly supplied with oxygen via the bloodstream. Normal breathing gives all the air the body cells need and maintains a steady flow of oxygen into the body. Exert that same body however, as in exercise, and it will naturally need more oxygen, necessitating a faster heart rate. That is the reason for the heart's speedup—it needs to feed more vital oxygen to the cells.

When this was discovered, it became necessary to find a way to measure how much oxygen is needed for various stages of exertion, that is, what is the body's aerobic capacity? To do that, the term *Met units* was devised, which are multiples of the body's resting energy requirements (e.g. two Mets require twice the resting energy cost, three Mets triple, etc.). This may sound complicated, but the following chart should clarify it. You will notice that each exercise or activity uses up a certain number of Mets, which in turn can be calculated at how many calories are burned up every minute. This chart gives you an assessment of the value of each particular exercise in inducing cardiovascular fitness.

Note: Energy range does vary depending on skill of exerciser, amount and pattern of rest pauses, environmental temperature, etc. Caloric values depend on body size (more for a larger person). The chart provides reasonable "relative strenuous values" however.

Energy range	Activity	Comment	Calories burned per hour
1.5–2.0 Mets	Light housework such as polishing furniture or washing small clothes.	Too low in energy level and too intermittent to promote endurance.	120–150
	Strolling 1 mile/hr.	Not sufficiently strenuous to promote endurance unless capacity is very low.	
2.0–3.0 Mets	Level walking at 2 miles/ hr.	See "strolling."	150–240
	Golf, using power cart.	Promotes skill and minimal strength in arm muscles but not sufficiently taxing to promote endurance. Also too intermittent.	
3.0–4.0 Mets	Cleaning windows, mopping floors or vacuuming	Adequate conditioning exercise if carried out continuously for 20–30 minutes.	240–300
	Bowling.	Too intermittent and not sufficiently taxing to promote endurance.	
	Walking 3 miles/hr.	Adequate dynamic exercise if low capacity.	
	Cycling 6 miles/hr.	As above.	
	Golf, pulling cart.	Useful for conditioning if reach target rate. May	

		include isometrics de-pending on cart weight.	
4.0–5.0 Mets	Scrubbing Floors.	Adequate endurance exercise if carried out in at least 2-minute stints.	300–360
	Walking 3.5 miles/hr.	Usually good dynamic aerobic exercise.	
	Cycling 8 miles/hr.	As above.	
	Table tennis, badminton and volleyball.	Vigorous continuous play can have endurance benefits but intermittent, easy play only promotes skill.	
	Golf, carrying clubs.	Promotes endurance if reach and maintain target heart rate; otherwise merely aids strength and skill.	
	Tennis, doubles.	Not very beneficial unless there is continuous play maintaining target rate, which is unlikely. Will aid skill.	
	Many calisthenics and ballet exercises.	Will promote endurance if continuous, rhythmic and repetitive. Those requiring isometric effort such as pushups and situps are probably not beneficial for cardiovascular fitness.	

5.0–6.0 Mets	Walking 4 miles/hr.	Dynamic, aerobic and of benefit.	360–420
	Cycling 10/miles hr.	As above.	
	Ice or roller skating.	As above is done continuously.	
6.0–7.0	Walking 5 miles/hr.	Dynamic, aerobic and beneficial.	420–480
	Cycling 11 miles/hr.	As above.	
	Singles tennis.	Can provide benefit if played 30 minutes or more by skilled player with an attempt to keep moving.	
	Water skiing.	Total isometrics; very risky for cardiacs, pre-cardiacs (high risk) or deconditioned normals.	
7.0–8.0 Mets	Jogging 5 miles/hr.	Dynamic, aerobic, endurance building exercise.	480–600
	Cycling 12 miles/hr.	As above.	
	Downhill skiing.	Usually ski runs are too short to significantly promote endurance. Lift may be isometric. Benefits skill predominantly. Combined stress of altitude, cold and exercise may be too great for some cardiacs.	

	Paddleball.	Not sufficiently continuous but promotes skill. Competition and hot playing areas may be dangerous to cardiacs.	
8.0–9.0 Mets	Running 5.5 miles/hr.	Excellent conditioner.	600–660
	Cycling 13 miles/hr.	As above.	
	Squash or handball (practice session or warm-up)	Usually too intermittent to provide endurance-building effect. Promotes skill.	
Above 10 Mets	Running 6 miles/hr = l0 Mets 7 miles/hr = 11.5 8 miles/hr = 13.5	Excellent conditioner.	660
	Competitive handball or squash.	Competitive environment in a hot room is dangerous to anyone not in excellent physical condition.	

Though it is impossible to determine an accurate aerobic level without first being examined by a doctor, the accompanying diagram will give you an indication of where you stand. Your capacity decreases as you get older, but as the target zone on the chart indicates, the benefits of rhythmic exercise apply to all ages.

How do you put that information to use? Remember that it is crucial to stay within the target zone at all times. Obviously, many people will be able to attain maximal aerobic capacity, but it is of little extra use in conditioning the heart and will only leave you breathless and unable to continue the

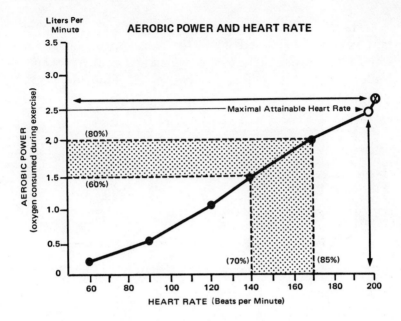

AEROBIC POWER AND HEART RATE

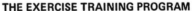

THE EXERCISE TRAINING PROGRAM

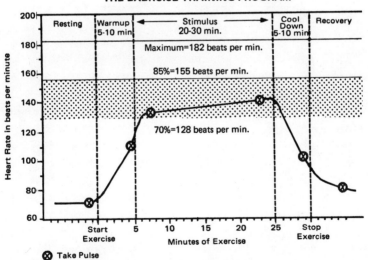

exercise. Playing safe is very much a ground rule that should be followed, if only to ensure that jogging, swimming etc., remain a pleasure to you.

The exercise training pattern gives you an indication of how your body responds from the warm-up period at the start of the exercise to the cool-down and recovery at the end. Your heart rate, you will see, never goes out of the safety gap.

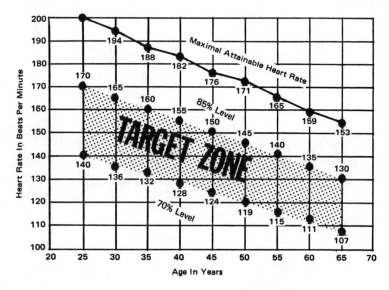

How can you tell whether you are staying within the safety gap? As a very general guide, you will know as soon as you have gotten into your exercise. You will be doing it with seemingly little effort and will genuinely feel that you can go on forever. With jogging, for instance, it is tempting to begin too fast and after less than a mile you will be completely out of breath. Try it slower and more gently and you will gradually grasp what you are trying to attain; the baffling mystery of the staying power of the long distance runner will be as clear to you as daylight.

To back up your first impressions of how you are performing, test your pulse to see if your heart rate matches the target zone determined for you during your initial checkup. To do this you can feel the pulse point at your wrist, neck, forehead or groin and check the beats against a watch with a second hand. The pulses normally beat at exactly the same rate as your heart, so if you prefer just feel the heart beats. You must do this immediately on stopping the exercise because in the five or ten minutes that follow you will recover and the heart will go back to beating at its normal level. It is not even necessary to feel the pulse for a whole minute. Count the beats in a ten-second period and then simply multiply them by six to get the heart rate per minute. If it is above the target range, tone down your exercise—which is common sense of course—and conversely, if it is below, you are not quite working at your target level and you need to exercise more strenuously.

Obviously if you have been sedentary for a long period of time your exercise will bring about aches and pains that are indicative of the body adjusting itself to a new life of activity. Most of the pains will be muscular, but it is well to know the danger signs of problems in the region of the heart if they should occur. The diagram on the following page will help you; also note the warnings that follow.

Warnings and What to Do About Them

Symptom	Cause	Remedy
STOP! See physician before resuming.		
1. Abnormal heart action; e.g., pulse becoming irregular; fluttering, jumping or palpitations in chest or throat; sudden bursts of rapid heart beats; sudden very slow pulse when a moment before it had been on target. (Immediate or delayed)	Extra heartbeats, dropped heartbeats or disorders of cardiac rhythm. This may or may not be dangerous and should be checked out by a physician.	Consult physician before resuming exercise program. You may have a harmless disorder or the physician may review your exercise program.

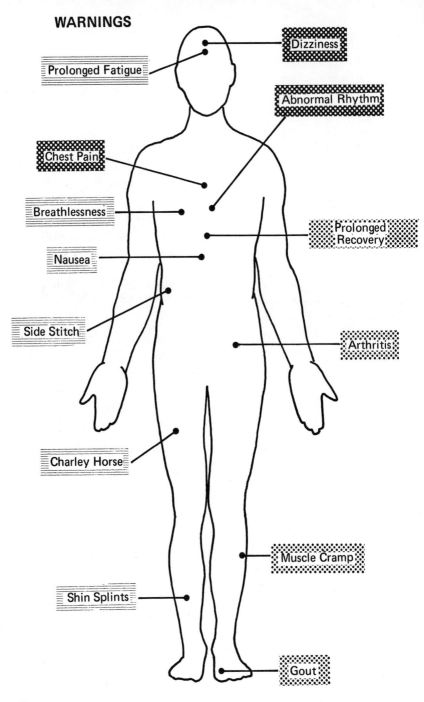

WARNINGS

Dizziness

Prolonged Fatigue

Abnormal Rhythm

Chest Pain

Breathlessness

Prolonged Recovery

Nausea

Side Stitch

Arthritis

Charley Horse

Muscle Cramp

Shin Splints

Gout

SEE YOUR PHYSICIAN OR DISCONTINUE EXERCISE PROGRAM

TRY SUGGESTED REMEDY BRIEFLY; SEE PHYSICIAN

YOU PROBABLY CAN HANDLE IT YOURSELF

2. Pain or pressure in the center of the chest or the arm or throat precipitated by or following exercise. (Immediate or delayed)	Possible heart pain.	Consult physician before resuming exercise.
3. Dizziness, lightheadedness, sudden incoordination, cold sweat, confusion, glassy stare, pallor, blueness or fainting. (Immediate)	Insufficient blood to the brain.	Do not try to cool down. Stop exercise and lie down with feet elevated, or put head down between legs until symptoms pass. Later, consult physician before next exercise session.

Remedies which may be self-administered.

4. Persistent rapid heart action near the target level even 5-10 minutes after the exercise was stopped. (Immediate)	Exercise is probably too vigorous.	Keep heart rate at lower end of target zone or below. Increase the vigor of exercise more slowly. If this does not control the excessively high recovery heart rate consult physician.
5. Flare-up of arthritic condition or gout which usually occurs in hips, knees, ankles or big toe — the weight-bearing joints. (Immediate or delayed)	Trauma to joints which are particularly vulnerable.	Rest up and do not resume your exercise program until condition subsides (using your usual remedies). Then resume exercise at a lower level with protective footwear on softer surfaces or select other exercises which will put less strain on joints.

Can be remedied without medical consultation.

6. Nausea or vomiting after exercise. (Immediate)	Not enough oxygen to the intestine. You are either exercising too vigorously or cooling down too quickly.	Exercise less vigorously and be sure to take a more gradual and longer cool-down.
7. Extreme breathlessness lasting more than 10 minutes after stopping exercise. (Immediate)	Exercise is too taxing to your cardiovascular system or lungs.	Stay at the lower end of your target range. If symptoms persist, do even less than target level. Be sure that while you are exercising you are not too breathless to talk to a companion.
8. Prolonged fatigue even 24 hrs. later. (Delayed)	Exercise is too vigorous.	Stay at lower end of your target range or below. Increase level more gradually.
9. Shin splints (pain on the front or sides of lower leg). (Delayed)	Inflammation of the fascia connecting the leg bones, or muscle tears where muscles of the lower leg connect to the bone.	Use shoes with thicker soles. Work out on turf, which is easier on your legs.
10. Insomnia which was not present prior to the exercise program. (Delayed)	Exercise is too vigorous.	Stay at lower end of target range or below. Increase intensity of exercise gradually.

11. Pain in the calf muscles which occurs on heavy exercise but not at rest. (Immediate)	May be due to muscle cramps due to lack of use of these muscles, or exercising on hard surfaces. May also be due to poor circulation to the legs (called claudication).	Use shoes with thicker soles, cool down adequately. Muscle cramps should clear up after a few sessions. If "muscle cramps" do not subside, circulation is probably faulty. Try another exercise; e.g., cycling instead of jogging in order to use different muscles.
12. Side stitch (sticking under the ribs while exercising). (Immediate)	Diaphragm spasm. The diaphragm is the large muscle which separates the chest from the abdomen.	Lean forward while sitting, attempting to push the abdominal organs up against the diaphragm.
13. Charley horse or muscle-bound feeling. (Immediate or delayed)	Muscles are deconditioned and unaccustomed to exercise.	Take hot bath. Next exercise should be less strenuous.

Holistic Tips:

- You must exercise to a certain intensity (which can be measured safely and accurately by heart rate) in order to gain the benefits of conditioning. For your own safety, do not exceed the heart rate prescribed by your doctor.
- Get a watch with a second hand that you can see easily. Turn the watch so that you can see it while you take your pulse rate. After you have been exercising steadily for 3-4 minutes, stop and immediately find your pulse and count the beats in the first 10

seconds. Multiply by six to get your pulse rate per minute.

- Each day, start by warming up for 5-10 minutes with moderate activity such as walking or calisthenics.
- Then exercise vigorously to maintain your target heart rate for at least 20 minutes. Every two weeks, increase the time by one minute as long as you are doing well. At about three months you will be exercising vigorously for 30 minutes or more each day. This should be continued as a lifelong pattern and will maintain your fitness at a high level.
- Cool off for 5-10 minutes with moderate activity such as walking.
- Your exercise will have to be gradually more strenuous in order to maintain your target heart rate. A slower heart rate is positive evidence of the benefit of exercise.
- Wear proper shoes that do not cause any discomfort during all exercises.
- Avoid fatigue, cramps, sore joints or discomfort of any kind.
- Take your time and enjoy yourself. Never push your program except to be regular and exercise every day.
- Remember that the best types of exercise are those that use both the arms and the legs.

After two or three weeks of regular exercise, you will begin to become aware of the benefits. If you were overweight, you might even begin to see those benefits in a flatter tummy, less fat on your legs, etc. Generally you will have gained an aura of well-being that will let you sleep better, refreshing you for the day ahead, and letting you approach your exercise routine with pleasure and ease, (and even a sense of disappointment if you should have to miss it for a day or two).

You will find that you can gradually elevate your aerobic capacity to allow you to run if you chose jogging, or jog if you chose walking. Again, you will keep on feeling that sense of effortless power until you reach your peak of physical fitness, just like any runner or other athlete. Once you get that far, you will have achieved the best conditioning for your heart, lungs and body. All your internal organs will function to their fullest. This, coupled with your new diet, will surely bring about a better life and one that is much freer from illness than ever before.

Next Time You Think You Are Dying
for a Cigarette... You May Be

If you are a smoker of cigarettes, cigars or a pipe, then you have a barrier to achieving full holistic health, because total well-being cannot be achieved with the hindrance of smoking. It has a detrimental effect both on physical fitness and the ability of your body to prevent disease. The advice of the holistic doctor is, therefore, the same as the advice of any physician. STOP. And that should not be next week, next month, or in a little while, but *now*. Unfortunately there is no other way, even if you believe you cannot function either at work or at leisure without the stimulation that tobacco smoking brings.

There is also danger for the nonsmoker if extended amounts of time are spent in the company of smokers. Research now shows that the constant inhalation of secondhand smoke poses considerable health hazards. These are in the form of allergic reactions or increased disposition to chronic illness caused, according to a 1978 report compiled by several leading health authorities (including two former surgeon generals of the U.S.), directly from the inhalation of substantial quantities of the 1150 chemical substances present in tobacco smoke.

In babies and young children, this effect is shown by studies carried out under Dr. J.R.T. Colley in England. He investigated the incidence of bronchitis and pneumonia in more than 2200 infants as it related to the smoking habits of their parents.

Dr. Colley also studied nearly 2500 six- to fourteen-year-olds and found that the prevalence of coughs was highest when both parents were smokers; intermediate when one parent was a smoker; and lowest when neither parent smoked.

In adults the issue is equally problematic. Dr. Frederick Speer of the University of Kansas Medical Center looked at the reactions of 400 nonsmokers subjected to levels of secondhand smoke in both working and social conditions. He found that over 70 percent suffered eye irritation; 46 percent reported headaches; while decreasing numbers complained of coughing, sore throats and nausea. Those findings are supported by New York pathologist Dr. Carl Becker, who contends that about one in every three people is allergic to tobacco whether or not a smoker. VA Hospital researchers in Long Beach, California, found that angina patients could expect increased pain if exposed to smoke for prolonged periods. Therefore, if you believe you are a "passive smoker," as secondhand smokers are known, then you would be well-advised to cut down your exposure either by helping the offenders quit smoking, or seeking a less polluted environment.

As for the smoker and holistic health, there is little that any doctor can say that is more convincing than the warning on the side of every pack of cigarettes. The evidence that links lung cancer, as well as heart disease and other chronic illnesses, to smoking is so heavily documented that only a fool would ignore it. Here is a way you can stop, without gadgets, pills or substitutes.

Begin by reviewing your cigarette routine. Consider when you smoke and tell yourself that it is possible to have a drink or drive to work without a cigarette. This will help you to switch your outlook to that of a nonsmoker. Then on the day you decide to quit, smoke right up until you finish work in the evening. Wait until the urge comes for another cigarette and then do something different like going for a walk. Breathe deeply and exhale, savoring the air around you. When the anxiety increases, go to bed early and sleep. When you awaken you will have gone perhaps 15 or 16 hours without a cigarette. Just think about that. It is almost the equivalent of a full waking day during which you could have smoked 30, 40, 50, or more, cigarettes. So having gone that long is a personal achievement. Now, with the right attitude, you are already on the way to conquering the habit.

On the second day, alter your routine. Skip breaks, walk at lunchtime, take public transportation instead of the car. In between times, nibble a few nuts or raisins to satisfy the craving for something in your mouth. Before long you will have doubled that 15 or 16 hours, and you can think in terms of making it 60 or 64 until to break your abstention would be a matter of personal honor. Convince yourself that you can be successful by thinking of the millions of people who go about their lives never giving a thought to smoking. Within a matter of a couple of weeks you no longer need be a slave to the little white stick, the craving will have disappeared, and you can begin a new way of life.

Above all, you will have done your body the greatest favor possible—and maybe even saved your life!

A POINT TO STRESS

It is just as important to know what kind of patient has a disease as what kind of disease a patient has.

The subject of cigarette smoking is an ideal introduction to the holistic health concept of stress and how to keep it under control, for in many cases, the cigarette will have been used as a stress reducer itself—a device to calm nerves during a crisis or as a comforter in times of depression. If you are a nonsmoker, you will have used something else in the same way. You will have consoled yourself with a bag of candy, calmed your nerves before a big occasion with a dash of spirits, or even turned to someone else for guidance on dealing with the crisis. Everyone at certain times has abnormal amounts of stress in his or her life and it is necessary to learn how to cope with it.

Some people cope very well with life's stresses. There are many businessmen and women who order their day so well that they can run five miles, be in the office by 9 a.m., make decisions all day long, have a dinner engagement, then rest—to start the whole thing all over again. Many of them live to a ripe old age, and still manage to keep on running. Business people are not the only ones. You probably know some sprightly old person who never ceases to amaze you. In many cases it is more by good luck than good management. These people have good constitutions and have, perhaps, remained active while eating a good diet that has appealed to their tastes. Others have been aware of the value of good nutrition, exercise, and relaxation, so that life and its illnesses are not a mystery to them. Thus they can control their bodies and their minds.

Coping with stress means learning to deal with the ordinary and the extraordinary pressures of your life. The inability to cope manifests itself in many ways. Holistic doctors find that people suffering from ulcers, headaches, hypertension, and various other chronic ailments as well as anxiety states, are having a problem with stress. Stress aggravates these illnesses via changes in the body chemistry which are not fully understood. The social consequences are enormous. Besides the pain and suffering, stress and stress-related illnesses cost money—an estimated 50 billion dollars each year as a result of heart disease and over 15 billion dollars as a result of alcoholism. Business has noted the effects in the form of lost workdays, excessive turnover and lower productivity. A New New York business magazine has cited estimates that 52 million persondays of production are lost annually. Less obvious costs include higher group insurance rates, more production errors, and diminished judgment on the part of key personnel. Holistic doctors and other physicians specializing in stress sometimes see it as job-related, but also note its link with marital relationships, family problems, money difficulties, social changes, and other emotional and spiritual considerations.

A certain amount of stress is good for us. Athletes need to experience stress in order to be in top form. Ordinary people utilize stress to perform difficult tasks, ensure quick reactions, be successful at examinations, or avoid a moment of danger. But as life for everyone has become much more complex, so have the stresses increased. How difficult they are to deal with depends on your type of personality. Each day we interact with our friends, peers, husbands, wives, children, teachers, employers or employees. They all demand something of us. In today's highly technological society it is easy to see why anxieties and pressures on our nervous system can soon get out of hand.

Stress, it seems, begins when the gap between our own reality and our own expectation grows too wide. One aim of holistic medicine is to train every patient to cope with day-to-day worries and try to remedy distorted expectations and realities. When stress is properly managed there is a definite improvement in the well-being of the individual.

The following questionnaire is based upon statistical evaluations of stressful situations and can actually predict your chances of a stress-related illness in the future. Mark off any that are relevant to your recent past and then consult the scoring comments following the list.

Stress Evaluator

	Event	Value
1.	Death of spouse	100
2.	Divorce	73
3.	Marital separation	65
4.	Jail term	63
5.	Death of close family member	63
6.	Personal injury or illness	53
7.	Marriage	50
8.	Fired from work	47
9.	Marital reconciliation	45
10.	Retirement	45
11.	Change in family member's health	44
12.	Pregnancy	40
13.	Sex difficulties	39
14.	Addition to family	39
15.	Business readjustment	39
16.	Change in financial status	38
17.	Death of a close friend	37
18.	Change to different line of work	36
19.	Change in number of marital arguments	35
20.	Mortgage or loan over $10,000	31
21.	Foreclosure of mortgage or loan	30
22.	Change in work responsibilities	29
23.	Son or daughter leaving home	29
24.	Trouble with in-laws	29
25.	Outstanding personal achievement	28
26.	Spouse begins or stops work	26
27.	Starting or finishing school	26
28.	Change in living conditions	25
29.	Revision of personal habits	24
30.	Trouble with boss	23
31.	Change in work hours, conditions	20
32.	Change in residence	20
33.	Change in schools	20
34.	Change in recreational habits	19

35. Change in church activities   19
36. Change in social activities   18
37. Mortgage or loan under $10,000   17
38. Change in sleeping habits   16
39. Change in number of family gatherings   15
40. Change in eating habits   15
41. Vacation   13
42. Christmas season   12
43. Minor violation of the law   11

(Based on the Social Readjustment Rating Scale developed by Thomas Holmes, M.D., of the University of Washington Medical School, with Richard Rahe.)

Your score is determined by adding up your total number of points. If you totalled up to 50, chances are you are not under much stress. From 50 to 150, problems are beginning to arise and you have a fair chance (in fact, a 37 percent chance), of getting a stress-related illness in the next twelve months. That percentage goes to 51 if your score is between 150 and 300; above 300, the sickness chances are 80 percent. These evaluations were made by questioning thousands of people about their life changes, but it must be emphasized that everybody is different. This should only be treated as a guide to whether you should consider beginning a stress management program.

Dr. Holmes says stress-related illness is now so widespread that it's more common than illness caused by germs. Nowadays germs are generally to blame for only minor diseases. Certainly medical researchers agree they are unlikely to have anything to do with the causation factors behind cancer, heart disease and most of the chronic illnesses. If dietary factors and a lack of exercise can be ruled out, then at the root of the problem could be a stress-related factor as diverse as the top and bottom of the scale. Interestingly, in support of this, a study of 5000 patients at New York Hospital showed that same diversity of incidents before the onset of the illness. Everyday events like a vacation were enough to trigger illnesses.

Stress Reduction

Learning about the workings of your own body helps in the management of stress. Holistic doctors sometimes teach patients about their bodies by a technique known as *biofeedback* which has had tremendous success in recent years. A series of monitoring instruments are connected by sensors to the patient's head and hands. Audible and visual signals reveal what is going on in the patient's body. Eventually, at will, he is able to trigger the signals or stop them. The patient learns to control his so-called autonomic body functions with his mind, and subsequently to control stress reactions in the same way.

Many other methods of stress reduction and management are used in holistic clinics, ranging from group therapy to hypnosis, massage, and even dance therapy. Holistic doctors have found these techniques work much better, and have many fewer potential problems associated with them, than anti-anxiety medication. After all, no doctor has ever yet diagnosed a Valium deficiency, and is not likely to in the foreseeable future.

It has also been observed by Dr. Carl Simonton, a medical oncologist, that a person's attitude towards their disease can exert some influence over its course. Patients generally do better if they have a stronger will to live and a more positive stance towards life. Part of the stress management and healing processes in holistic clinics is geared towards that outlook, motivating the patient and his beliefs in a positive direction, keeping hopes, memories and realities in their proper perspective.

Once that has been mastered, any patient has taken a giant step in the process of self-healing and prevention of illness.

The Road Ahead

Few people are unaware of the fads and fancies that have moved the American people in the last decade or so. Early on there came "flower power" with which we all suddenly saw the beauties of our fertile soil while liberated songsters sang of love, not war. Then the hippies "discovered" meditation and sat down with the Beatles to find themselves within, rather than without. The peace movement gathered momentum and all of a sudden there was a new band of veterans from yet another war. Transactional Analysis really made it big and existentialism did quite well too, while yoga ticked steadily through it all, until lately, when awareness and consciousness and charismatic renewal occupy the minds of many. Some of those, of course, have much validity in the meaning of life, while others will be as forgettable as yesterday's newspapers. The point about them all is that they were, and are, signs of the people striving for something above themselves. There has been a basic realization that science and technology do not have all the answers to health and wellness, and it is this that has turned the wheels of the holistic movement. It is not another fad or fancy because keeping well and healthy is much more deeply rooted in our very existence than in technological advancement.

Man is frustrated with technology, big business and goverment being unable to deal with people on a humanistic level. People are tired of being a number or a commodity for profit; tired of getting into a hospital with white walls, plastic furniture and X-ray machines harmful to health; tired of having fingers stuck in his nose and ear while the rest of his body is ignored. The idealism of one ailment, one pill, one cure, just doesn't work. New drugs, new vaccines and more sophisticated surgery is not the answer.

Holistic medicine has a greater sense of humanism and a greater sense of what we need to survive. It is also true that many doctors are tired of breaking people down into parts and numbers, but they are inexorably caught up in a system to which they must pay allegiance, because it was they who originally formulated it. Holistic doctors have broken away and are being sought because there are growing numbers of people looking for the total approach. Together they have started a new age in which health care will not be dictated by a drug-oriented mechanistic philosophy.

It is gratifying to note that changes within the medical establishment are beginning to occur. In 1978 Dr. Lester Breslow and Associates of the University of California at Los Angeles pointed out seven basic and simple changes which, if observed, would increase life expectancy.

These changes are:
• Eat three regular meals daily and no in-between-meal snacks.
• Eat breakfast.
• Keep body weight in the normal range.
• Get regular physical exercise.
• Get seven to eight hours of sleep daily.
• Do not smoke.
• Limit alcohol intake to not more than two drinks daily.

It has been estimated that men at age 45 who follow six or seven of these health-related behaviors can expect to live, on the average, until age 78. This is an eleven-year increase of life expectancy to be achieved merely by a few simple life-style changes. With three or fewer of these behavior changes, death would be expected at only 67 years.

The greatest healer is not the American health-care system, but ourselves. Billions of dollars have been spent on technological medicine, yet, as we know, life expectancy has barely changed. That will not come until the realization is nationwide that we *can* prevent the diseases that plague our society.

For many years the American Medical Association has been one of the cornerstones of the health-care system in the U.S.; it is an organization of physicians only. Now, in order to provide a sound springboard for the holistic movement, the American Holistic Medical Association has been formed and it is something of a milestone. It is also composed of traditional physicians—not herbalists, naturopaths or other practitioners without medical training—who are beginning to recognize the benefits of treating people with *more* than drugs and scientific instruments. With the AHMA, doctors have banded together to define what holistic medicine is and how it can be developed.

When the association was formed at an inaugural meeting in Denver, the number of holistically inclined doctors throughout the country was estimated to be about 3000— only a small minority of physicians. But there is evidence that those numbers are growing rapidly. Patients should be aware, however, that many self-styled practitioners are giving so-called holistic treatment without being properly trained in medicine. Most doctors believe that in order to provide a true medical clinic there should be at least one physician operating there. Therefore, people going for holistic treatment should check that the doctor does belong to an organization like the AHMA. If the physician does not have this affiliation, it could be that he is misrepresenting himself in his capacity as a doctor. It is a good check to make and one that will ensure your receiving all the benefits growing out of the holistic medicine movement.

As to the future of the HMG, it will be working towards a much greater and broader acceptance of the concept of holistic health. One of those targets will be the insurance companies. In general, the third-party carriers have not yet recognized the value of preventive medicine. But we believe they will once people demand it; and patients who have received the benefits of holistic medicine should begin to apply public pressure now. They must do this by lobbying Congressmen, Senators, and politicians at all levels. They should demand that the health-care dollars of this country be spent on patient education and preventive processes so that the incidence of chronic diseases may be reduced.

The time has come to make a stand and to demand quality control of health care services. With the present trend, the cost of insurance premiums will go higher and higher until you refuse to pay. If that happens, the crisis point will occur and the system will go bankrupt; that is, unless the government, insurance companies, and doctors orient themselves to preventive medicine.

The government is already getting the message. Special probes into health care in recent years that span both spending and preventive medicine have reached the Surgeon General. But there are many outside influences that attempt to dissuade the govenment from taking wholesale measures to change. Not the least are the drug companies that dominate the system. Their entire economy is based on disease, for if there were none, there would be no need for the products they provide.

As things are now, however, they are among the biggest profit-makers in the world, and it cannot be overstated that the drug companies are a powerful group and it is in their interest that the people "need" and be prescribed their products. If you keep on taking their pills, they make money. This can only change when doctors and patients are shown other ways.

Holistic patients have been markedly able to control

their use of drugs. A further shift in public opinion would
shake the ground under the giants' feet and convince all the
top power manipulators that they rely on your dollars, and
yours alone.

The medical schools must also recognize that there is an
alternative to prescribing pills. They must convince the drug
companies that there is a future in preventive medicine and
that people must take precedence over profits. Time too must
be given over to young men and women starting out to become doctors, to educate them on the effects of pollution, refined food, chemical additives, lack of exercise and unnecessary surgical treatments. There will be no long-term prevention of disease until it is realized at all levels that man and his
environment are one and the same. Man will be what his environment is, and if that is polluted, then he will be too.

As we march on in the name of progress, our industries,
wastes, insecticides, automobiles, polluted tap water and our
lifestyles are making us sicker and sicker. We must all demand that our food be left free of insecticides, unrefined, un-
colored, and unflavored. We must all demand to know when
our water and the air we breathe will be improved, and our
haste and greed for progress slowed. Until we recognize that
everything as a convenience is not advancement in our society, but a detriment, we can only edge nearer and nearer to
social catastrophe with our growing susceptibility to chronic
illness.

Yet for all the problems we face, and for all the battles
we must fight to force changes in a seemingly irrevocable
system, it would not be appropriate to end this account of
the philosophy and practices of holistic health on a low
and disconsolate note. For there is hope of a new outlook,
as indicated in the ongoing studies and patient testimonials
in support of preventive medicine, many of which have
been quoted here. It is fitting therefore, to conclude with
the views of those who comprise, after all, the entire
medical equation—doctor and patient. All the follow-

ing, we believe, perfectly capture the mood of these changing times. The physician is Dr. Irvin Page of the internationally famous Cleveland Clinic, who told the sixty-second annual scientific assembly of the Interstate Postgraduate Medical Association in Hollywood, Florida:

> Medicine has undergone a revolution in the last fifty years. The pendulum has swung from the art of medicine to the science; and now it is swinging back.
>
> The good physician is able to combine the two in practice, using intuition and common sense.
>
> The lack of absolute right and wrongs in medicine has created a troubled zone that is now attracting public and governmental attention.
>
> Physicians must acknowledge the revolution and resolve to set an example of freedom used in its best sense. A moral and ethical democracy is within our grasp—we only have to reach out for it.

Addendum: Patients' Forum

Hypoglycemia

"Having now been informed about hypoglycemia, in looking back I can clearly see where it all started with me. My maternal grandmother had always been big on sweets. She loved her tea-and-sweets breaks at 10 a.m. and 3 p.m. each day, until she developed diabetes, of which she died at a young age of 62. It was easy to see how my mother would naturally love her sweets as well; chocolate was her favorite. She would eat a piece of chocolate first thing in the morning upon rising. I got into the same habit. At 10 a.m. and 3 p.m. every day we had our tea breaks too, along with sweets. We had sweets after dinner too. And in our lunches at school. My mom spent a fortune on candy bars. In other words, I grew up on sugar. I even ate chocolate in the middle of the night (kept in my nightstand). I craved sweets all the time.

In high school I had my first experience in getting so hungry and sick to my stomach and lightheaded that I would pass out . . . at around 3 p.m. I had always been sluggish, tired, sleepy, and generally always depressed. I was always crying for no reason. When I got older and was married, I was always depressed, crying, irritable, tired, had temper tantrums and was generally an emotionally unstable person. I went to doctors at two hospitals and asked them, 'What's wrong with me?' They answered, 'Not a thing—it's in your head.' Sometimes I wouldn't be able to go back to sleep after waking at night.

Most of the time I had to take Valium to get to sleep. It became a habit to take a couple before bed. I couldn't think straight anymore. I went to a couple more doctors about my problems and they prescribed pills for my nerves. I felt that suicide was the only answer. It was at this point when my teacher from church, concerned about my depression, came by and told me it sounded as if I had hypoglycemia. He had it. He gave me the name of a holistic health doctor. Holistic health is a godsend to me. It has changed my life. My entire attitude to life is different—as long as I stay away from sweets and sugar. When I do snitch, I get really sick and all my old symptoms come back. I feel the Lord brought me and holistic medicine together to save my life."

Housewife—Mrs. I. H.

Stress

"My experience of learning to apply the principles of holistic medicine was as though I had stepped out of a dark and painful tunnel, into the light of self-awareness and healing. After growing up and trying to fulfill the American Dream—marriage and children—I failed. Divorced at 22 and the mother of a two-year-old daughter. She was gorgeous, a dream come true, but I had to raise her on my own. We moved into a little cottage. I got a job at a nice department store, and we began to live on our own.

All too quickly our dream of independence was shattered. I couldn't make it. I didn't feel well and I was beginning to get more and more withdrawn from the world and my family. I was going crazy and was falling apart from anxiety. I just couldn't show strength enough to be on my own. One morning, not too much later, I woke up in the intensive-care unit at county hospital. I had tried to commit suicide and failed, and had been unconscious for five days. Then came the HMG.

What is happening to me now is a therapy that is strengthening my body's defense mechanisms. To reduce my stress, which was being brought on by bad diet and environmment, causing toxic poisons to flow throughout my blood stream, I'm being guided through procedures necessary to rule out the chances of any more degeneration. I'm learning all about nutrition, vitamins and a balance of what my body needs to maintain a healthy normal existence. I've quit smoking a pack of cigarettes a day, taken the chemicals out of my home, changed to Ivory soap, no more perfumes or sprays of any kind, and anything else that I could do to complete my part. By applying the simple principles of holistic medicine I have been met halfway in my quest for healing."

Housewife—Mrs. D. R.

Allergies/Hypoglycemia

"Several years ago when I was working 60 hours per week, it did not concern me when I would periodically get very tired and sleep 14-16 hours. I figured my body needed the rest. However, when I slowed down to a normal work week and still had the same fatigue, I became concerned, so I told my doctor. He said: 'Don't worry about it. Since your job permits, go ahead and take a nap when you get tired.' With a pat on the head and a bottle of pills, I went home, only to return a year later with the same complaint. Another round of tests and nothing wrong could be found. I insisted there was something wrong so the doctor referred me to an internist. The internist referred me to a psychiatrist. The psychiatrist said I was cyclothymic (a mild form of manic-depressive). He prescribed Vivoctal for depression which I took for over a year. I began working shorter days and fewer days. I would go home tired, often too tired and fatigued to even answer the phone. When I became so low that I had only worked a few days in a month, I went to a holistic doctor who diagnosed hypoglycemia with multiple-food allergies and a deficiency in several vitamins and minerals.

Within three weeks, I felt better than I could remember feeling in six years. As I learned more, I realized I have had intermittently many symptoms as long as twenty years ago. Every day I feel better than the day before. There is no doubt that I am healthier, happier, have more vigor and stamina and will soon be richer from having gone to a holistic doctor."

Realtor—Mr. J.P.

Nutrition

"My grandparents were farmers in Germany. I grew up eating a very simple, healthy diet: whole grains, fresh fruits, lots of vegetables, very little fish or meat and no added salt. When I came to this country in 1958, I began to eat the typical American diet, high in meat and refined, processed foods, with the following results: my first cavity at 27; varicose veins and hemorrhoids by the age of 35; large brown 'liver' spots on my face since 1963; constant problems with fever blisters, sores in my mouth, and yeast infections. I was always tired, and fought an unending battle against obesity.

Then, a friend brought the growing body of literature on nutrition and healthful living to my attention. We began to take vitamin and mineral supplements and shop in health food stores. We studied books and magazines avidly for new information. Our health did improve. That improvement is best illustrated by my reactions to two similar operations. Several years before I became interested in nutrition, the veins were stripped from my right leg because of the danger of blood clots. The same operation was performed on my left leg in 1972. After the first operation, I was in great pain for a week. I stayed in the hospital for nine days. After the second operation, I had no pain. I was walking 30 minutes after I left the recovery room. I left the hospital the next day. Even with this vast improvement, I still had problems. I continued to have a number of minor infections, the brown spots remained in my face, and my weight was still hard to control. I had periods of nausea and dizziness. We kept searching for the answers to these problems.

We moved to California where we discovered a holistic doctor who performed a series of tests that identified that I had low blood sugar, some food and chemical allergies, some mineral deficiencies, and an almost total lack of hydrochloric acid. I was put on an immediate juice fast which helped me work out changes in my diet and environment. I loved the juice fast and extended it from one to two weeks. I had immediate relief from long-standing gas and bloating. The nausea and dizziness did not recur. I felt better than I ever had in my life. I'm following the diet and changing my lifestyle. My hypoglycemia is under control. I've had no cold sores or infections for months. The dark brown 'liver' spots visible in my face for fifteen years have almost disappeared. I've lost fifteen pounds and I feel marvelous."

Housewife—Mrs. T.B.

General Bibliography

Blaine, Tom R. *Goodbye Allergies*. Secaucus, NJ: Citadel Press, 1968.

Cheraskin, Emanuel, et al. *Diet and Disease*. Emmaus, PA: Rodale Press, 1968.

———*Psycho-dietetics*. New York: Stein and Day, 1974.

Coca, Arthur. *Pulse Test*. New York: Arc Books, 1968.

Dickey, Lawrence D. *Clinical Ecology*. Springfield, IL: C. C. Thomas, 1976.

Galos, Natalie. *Management of Complex Allergies*. Send check for $11.50 to N.E. Foundation for Allergic Environmental Diseases, 3 Brush St., Norwalk, CT 06850.

Harper, Harold W. and Michael Culbert. *How You Can Beat the Killer Diseases*. New Rochelle, NY: Arlington House, 1978.

Kirschmann, John D. and Nutrition Search, Inc. *Nutrition Almanac*. New York: McGraw-Hill, 1975.

Leonard, Jon et al. *Live Longer Now*. New York: Grosset & Dunlap, 1974.

Leonard, Jon and Elaine Taylor. *Live Longer Now Cookbook*. New York: Grosset & Dunlap, 1977.

Mackarness, Richard. *Eating Dangerously: The Hazards of Hidden Allergies*. New York: Harcourt Brace Jovanovich, 1976.

Newbold, H. L. *Mega-Nutrients for Your Nerves*. New York: Wyden Books, 1975.

Passwater, Richard. *Super Nutrition*. New York: Dial, 1975.

Randolph, Theron G. *Human Ecology and Susceptibility to the Chemical Environment*. Springfield, IL: C.C. Thomas, 1976.

Roth, June. The *The Food-Depression Connection*. Chicago: Contemporary Books, 1978.

Selye, Hans. *The Stress of Life*. rev. ed. New York: McGraw-Hill, 1976.

Taube, E. Louis, M.D. *Food Allergy and the Allergic Patient*. Springfield, IL: C. C. Thomas, 1973.

Williams, Roger J. *Biochemical Individuality*. Austin: University of Texas Press, 1969.

———*Nutrition Against Disease*. New York: Bantam, 1973.

———*Nutrition in a Nutshell*. New York: Dolphin, 1962.

The Authors . . . .

Richard Kaplan, D.O., a native of New Jersey, is a graduate of Franklin and Marshall College and the Kansas City College of Osteopathic Medicine. He served as Chief Medical Officer at the U.S. Coast Guard Air Station at Miami, Florida, attaining the rank of Lieutenant Commander.

He left a general practice in Hollywood, Florida to join the Holistic Medical Group in 1977. Dr. Kaplan is a charter member of the American Holistic Medical Association; a member of the American Osteopathic Association; the International Academy of Preventive Medicine; the Orthomolecular Society; the American Academy of Medical Preventics; the San Francisco Vegetarian Society and the Collaborative Health Program of the San Francisco Consortium. He is married and lives in Berkeley, California.

Barry Saltzman, D.O., a native of New York, is a graduate of Adelphi University and the Kansas City College of Osteopathic Medicine. Dr. Saltzman is the founder of the Student Osteopathic Medical Association; clinical instructor of Family Practice at the University of California, Davis; a founder of the American Holistic Medical Association; a member of the Osteopathic Physicians and Surgeons of California; the International Academy of Preventive Medicine and the American Academy of Medical Preventics.

Dr. Saltzman is married to Marietta Guinta, a dance therapist, and they live with their two children in Tiburon, California.

Laurence Ecker, D.O., a native of Pennsylvania, is a graduate of Rutgers University and the College of Osteopathic Medicine and Surgery. Dr. Ecker is a charter member of the American Holistic Medical Association; the Orthomolecular Society; the American Osteopathic Association; the American Academy of Medical Preventics; the Osteopathic Physicians and Surgeons of California and the International

Academy of Preventive Medicine. He joined the Holistic Medical Group in 1976, and lives in Berkeley, California.

Patrick Wilkins is a British journalist now living in San Francisco, California.

THE OSTEOPATHIC PHYSICIAN (D.O.)

He is a qualified doctor, just like his colleague with the more familiar "M.D." after his name. He has gone through the same four-year graduate program with basically the same medical schooling.

Once awarded his degree, he has to pass an equivalent state license examination in order to practice.

He works in hospitals, clinics or family practice, and is able to prescribe the same therapies and medications in exactly the same way as his M.D. counterpart.

The difference lies in the way he sees his patients—as a whole, not just a person with a disease that needs fighting.

In 1874, a country doctor from Missouri, Andrew Taylor Still, M.D., decided that all the body's systems—the nerves, the circulation, the muscles and the bones—were interdependent and if one becomes ill, the others had their functions altered, too.

Thus osteopathy was born, and today some 16,000 D.O.s practice throughout the United States.

In many disorders, particularly of the back and spinal column, the D.O. offers something more than the M.D. in his treatment of the patient's symptoms.

Using the same system's interdependence knowledge, he is able to manipulate muscles, joints, nerves and bones to relieve pain, improve blood flow and stimulate the body's own illness-fighting mechanisms.

Holistic Health was the next logical step for many osteopathic doctors. We feel our osteopathic training is relevant to holistic medicine and it has been fully incorporated in our practice at the clinics.

Holistic Medical Group
Preventive & Nutritional Medicine
Family Practice
Allergy

3031 Tisch Way
San Jose, CA 95128
(408) 249-1991

935 Trancas St., Suite G
Napa, CA 94558
(707) 255-6800

4460 Redwood Highway
San Rafael, CA 94903
(415) 472-2343

1900 Mowry Ave., Suite 309
Fremont, CA 94536
(415) 797-3644

777 Southland Drive, Suite 210
Hayward, CA 94545
(415) 783-4600

211 Professional Bldg.
El Cerrito Plaza
El Cerrito, CA 94530
(415) 527-7020

1111 "A" St.
Antioch, CA 94509
(415) 757-4141

140 Joralemon St.
Brooklyn, NY 11201
(212) 624-1975